Dyscalculia

Dyscalculia is caused by developmental differences in the structures and patterns of activation in the brain. Affected learners require timely and tailored interventions, informed and shaped by neurological findings.

In this ground-breaking text, Professor Butterworth explains the latest research in the science of dyscalculia in a clear, non-technical way. Crucially, he shows that dyscalculia is caused by a core deficit in the ability to accurately and swiftly represent the number of objects in a set, an ability that underpins learning arithmetic, and clearly differentiates dyscalculia from other forms of early mathematical learning difficulties. Butterworth uniquely links research to pedagogical practice, to explain how science can be used for the identification of dyscalculia, and for the development of strategies to best help affected learners acquire arithmetical competence. The text provides robust interventions that focus on helping pupils to strengthen their ability to process numerosities and link them to the familiar number symbols, counting words and digits. It shows that science has clear and specific implications both for assessment and intervention.

A landmark publication for the dyscalculia community, *Dyscalculia: From Science to Education* will become an essential resource for teachers, professionals, parents and sufferers, as well as for university courses that include specific learning disabilities.

Brian Butterworth is Emeritus Professor of cognitive neuropsychology at the Institute of Cognitive Neuroscience at University College London, UK.

Dyscalculia
From Science to Education

Brian Butterworth

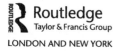
Routledge
Taylor & Francis Group

LONDON AND NEW YORK

First published 2019
by Routledge
2 Park Square, Milton Park, Abingdon, Oxon OX14 4RN

and by Routledge
52 Vanderbilt Avenue, New York, NY 10017

Routledge is an imprint of the Taylor & Francis Group, an informa business

British Library Cataloguing-in-Publication Data
A catalogue record for this book is available from the British Library

Library of Congress Cataloging-in-Publication Data
Names: Butterworth, Brian, author.
Title: Dyscalculia: from science to education / Brian Butterworth.
Description: Abingdon, Oxon; New York, NY: Routledge, 2019. |
Includes bibliographical references.
Identifiers: LCCN 2018033493 (print) | LCCN 2018046254 (ebook) |
ISBN 9781315538112 (eb) | ISBN 9781138688605 (hb) |
ISBN 9781138688612 (pb) | ISBN 9781315538112 (ebk)
Subjects: LCSH: Acalculia in children. | Special education—Mathematics. |
Mathematics—Study and teaching.
Classification: LCC RJ496.A25 (ebook) |
LCC RJ496.A25 B88 2019 (print) | DDC 618.92/85889—dc23
LC record available at https://lccn.loc.gov/2018033493

ISBN: 978-1-138-68860-5 (hbk)
ISBN: 978-1-138-68861-2 (pbk)
ISBN: 978-1-315-53811-2 (ebk)

Typeset in Bembo and Helvetica Neue
by codeMantra

Contents

Preface

In 2008, the UK Government Office for Science published a massive, authoritative and carefully-researched report, the *Foresight Mental Capital and Wellbeing Project* subtitled *Making the Most of Ourselves in the 21st Century*. It was led by a very distinguished board of scientists, and the government's Chief Scientific Officer, Sir John Beddington, who wrote:

> The Project's scope is possibly unparalleled. It has taken an independent look at the best available scientific and other evidence and has considered the factors that influence an individual's mental development and wellbeing from conception until death. It has assessed how these are affected by: the policies of key Government departments; by important stakeholders such as educators, healthcare professionals and employers; and by the diverse environments in which we live – families, communities and our physical surroundings. It has also analysed possible interventions to address the future challenges, drawing upon considerations such as scientific efficacy, economics, governance and ethics.

I contributed a chapter on dyscalculia, then a little-known and even less regarded, handicap. The Executive Summary made the following recommendation:

> Developmental dyscalculia – because of its low profile but high impacts, its priority should be raised. Dyscalculia relates to numeracy and affects between 4–7% of children. It has a much lower profile than dyslexia but can also have substantial impacts: it can reduce lifetime earnings by £114,000 and reduce the probability of achieving five or more GCSEs (A*–C) by 7–20 percentage points. Home and school interventions have again been identified by the Project. Also, technological interventions are extremely promising, offering individualised instruction and help, although these need more development.

The Labour government then asked Brian Lamb to carry out an inquiry into special educational needs. His report said a lot about dyslexia and autism, and made 51 recommendations, but it said nothing about dyscalculia, or even special educational needs in maths.

Needless to say, subsequent Conservative governments have done little or nothing to implement the recommendation from the Mental Capital report. Essentially, they have washed their hands of the problem. If you look on the Department for Education website, the only references to dyscalculia are that it will not prevent you getting a driving licence, and employers shouldn't discriminate against dyscalculics.

Despite official neglect, dyscalculia and maths learning difficulties have received much more attention since 2008. There are helpful websites; the British Dyslexia Association now recognises it as a handicap distinct from dyslexia and is starting courses to qualify teachers of dyscalculic learners. There are now many books about dyscalculia. Some are personal accounts of sufferers (Abeel, 2007; Moorcraft, 2014). There are guides for special needs teachers by special needs teachers (e.g. Adlam, 2012; Attwood & Bird, 2007; Chinn, 2007; Emerson & Babtie, 2013; Emerson & Babtie, 2014; Babtie & Emerson, 2015; Henderson, 2012; Hornigold, 2015).

So why am I writing another book about dyscalculia? Personal stories do not give the scientific background. Teaching guides by experienced teachers can provide valuable insights into methods that work with some children, and occasionally methods that don't work. Of course, teachers have to help whichever children they are required to teach, and, if they specialize in maths difficulties, they will have to deal with children selected by class teachers or parents as not achieving at the expected level. Now, this will include a wide variety of learners. Some may have behavioural problems, autism, dyslexia, ADHD, even undetected vision or hearing problems, and so on. All of these conditions are frequently, but not invariably, associated with maths difficulties. However, books by teachers do not explain *why* some learners just don't get numbers. Experienced and reflective practitioners can often identify dyscalculics – even if they have never heard the word or know about the condition – and find effective ways of helping them. However, this does not mean they are able to formulate a set of criteria that can help other teachers identify and help other dyscalculic learners. Nor should they be expected to do so. This is the job of scientists, and the *science of dyscalculia* is, finally, moving very fast. More than a hundred scientific papers have been published in the past five years. You really need to be a scientist working in the field even to hope to keep up, and to make a proper evaluation of the quality and implications of the published studies.

It is really important to understand the different causes of poor mathematical development, otherwise parents, teachers and other professionals, run the risk of treating all low attainers in the same way, and this won't help the learners or indeed the teachers. One size does not fit all. Dyscalculia is one cause of low attainment in numeracy, just as dyslexia is one cause of low attainment in literacy.

But to identify dyscalculic learners and design the appropriate interventions, it is necessary to have a systematic procedure to distinguish them from other low attainers, and this should be the starting point for designing a specific intervention for each learner.

Now it would be easy for me to provide a simple test, a *check list* of factors and symptoms, and a set of recommendations, so that the educational psychologist could carry out a "differential diagnosis" and propose a pre-determined set of intervention exercises. I will do this at the end of the book.

However, in my judgment and in my experience, it is vastly better that everyone concerned with the dyscalculic learner, including the learner, *understands* what the underlying problem is. Everyone is different, of course, and every learner comes to acquiring arithmetical competence with a unique set of cognitive abilities, and disabilities, a unique learning history, and particular anxieties and motivations. Skilled and reflective practitioners know this, and are able to adapt their assessments and interventions accordingly, but this is because they understand the learner's problems, partly through their professional training and partly from experience. The problem with dyscalculia is that there is almost never any professional training. Even at UCL – where I work – the doctoral course in educational psychology had one lecture on dyscalculia. No teacher I have spoken with has encountered dyscalculia in teacher training. This book is an attempt to fill that gap.

It's called *Dyscalculia: From Science to Education* because science underpins my approach to both the assessment of dyscalculia and how best to help the suffering learner. The science, needless to say, is complex. I have found it useful to think of the scientific studies in terms of the *causal modelling framework* proposed by Morton & Frith (1995). This comprises four levels of explanation for an individual or for a group, all of which may interact with the environment (see Figure I.1). For the environmental factors, I have included only those that involve education, formal and informal. However, many other environmental factors can play a role, including nutrition (especially inadequate nutrition), trauma, poverty, and birth difficulties. These factors can have effect at any or all of the levels of function, including the genetic, since gene expression can be modified by environmental factors.

The problem with many accounts of dyscalculia (whatever it's called, and, as we shall see, it's called by many different names) is that they start and end with the top level of explanation: individual differences in behaviour, in particular, individual differences in performance on standardized tests of arithmetic. Dyscalculia (or other terms that refer to mathematical disability) is defined by performance below an arbitrary cut-off – for example, the bottom 10%, or the bottom 6% (for example in the UK's *Numbers Count* project (Dowrick, 2015)), or some other level defined statistically. What these accounts do not do is go down to the next level to try to understand the cognitive causes of *why* the learner is in the bottom 10% or whatever (in fact, this is exactly what the *Numbers Count* project fails to do, and as we shall see in Chapter 10 on intervention, why many children fall through its intervention net).

But don't be put off. The story I will tell is a very simple one, despite the complications. Developmental dyscalculia, I will argue, is due to a *core deficit* in "domain-specific cognitive capacities" – that is, those capacities that are specific to processing numbers – in what I have called the *number module*. I will show that this deficit easy to identify in assessments, and has very straightforward implications for intervention. Further, we can identify abnormalities in the domain-specific brain network that supports number processing. We also have reason to believe that the condition is congenital – you are unlucky enough to be born with it. This does not mean that *all* developmental dyscalculics *inherit* the condition. Some will, since we know that it can run in families and that identical twins are likely both to have the same level of numerical abilities. Nevertheless, environmental factors, such as prematurity and birth trauma, can affect the relevant brain network from birth.

I have called this "developmental dyscalculia" to distinguish it from "acquired dyscalculia" (sometimes called "acalculia") which is due to damage to an otherwise typically developed mathematical brain, caused by injury, stroke, or disease. However, I will refer to developmental dyscalculia simply as *dyscalculia* in this book, and I deal with this acquired dyscalculia in a separate chapter, since its causes and presentations are quite different.

Although the book is called *Dyscalculia: From Science to Education*, I have tried to make the science accessible to readers without a scientific training. Technical terms are explained as I go along, as are interpretations of the scientific results.

LEVEL OF EXPLANATION	MEASURES	EDUCATIONAL CONTEXT
BEHAVIOURAL	Number sense Chapter 2	Society, school, and home Chapter 8
COGNITIVE	Starter kit for learning arithmetic Chapter 3 Core deficit as the cause of dyscalculia Chapter 4	Assessment Chapter 9
	Development of arithmetic Chapter 5	Intervention Chapter 10
NEURAL	Brain structures and functions Chapter 6	Policy Chapter 11
	GENETIC AND OTHER CAUSES Chapter 7	

Figure I.1 Schematic model of the relationships among levels of explanation – genetic, neural, cognitive, and behavioural – following the causal modelling framework. A domain-general cognitive capacity and a domain-specific cognitive capacity can have effects on more than one behavioural test, and performance on a behavioural test may be affected by more than one cognitive capacity. Moreover, one cognitive capacity may depend on another (e.g., memory on attention), and one behaviour may causally affect another (e.g., poor reading may impair mathematical problem solving). Environment, and specifically educational context, can affect all capacities.

Because this book is based on the rapidly expanding science of dyscalculia, there will be disagreements among scientists about theory and evidence.

It would be easy enough to present only evidence or arguments that support my hypothesis that dyscalculia is caused by a core deficit in the number module, but this would misrepresent the current state of the science. So, I will point out these disagreements, and the extent to which they support or modify the story I am telling. I will try to reference all the relevant studies, though I am well aware that many readers will not have easy access to the technical literature, nor indeed an interest in reading it. Nevertheless, I provide these references for readers who are interested. On the whole, I don't believe that the disagreements affect how best to identify dyscalculia and how best to help dyscalculic sufferers.

I am often told by educationalists that it is bad to "label" people. All the dyscalculics I have worked with tell me that it is far, far better to be labelled dyscalculic than to be labelled stupid, not only because of the ways others see them, but, perhaps more importantly, how they see themselves.

Science is a collaborative enterprise, and my work on dyscalculia is no exception. I couldn't have done any of the work described in this book without the help of many people – students, post-docs, senior colleagues, lab visitors, and members of two European networks I coordinated, *Neuromath* and *Numbra*. Three particular events set me on the path to dyscalculia. First, I met Carlo Semenza, a young Italian doctor, psychologist, psychiatrist, psychoanalyst, and cook, at a meeting on our joint interest at that time, aphasia – the effects of brain damage on speech and language. We decided to take advantage of two EU initiatives, both now at risk: the Erasmus programme for exchanging students, and a scheme for funding cooperative research.

Through this I met one of Carlo's brilliant Italian students, Lisa Cipolotti, who said she wanted to do a doctorate with me in London on aphasia. However, when she got here, she changed her mind, and decided she wanted to do something new in neuropsychology, something no-one or at least very few people, were researching. I thought that acquired dyscalculia would fill the bill. I knew a bit about it because I had been interested in the foundations of mathematics – though from a logical rather than an empirical point of view. A little research showed that, back in 1989, one could read the entire literature in two weeks, and that only one person was actively working in this area, and that was my colleague, Elizabeth Warrington. We discovered – perhaps re-discovered would be a better term – that the damage to the left parietal lobe in the brain routinely led to difficulties even with very simple numerical tasks.

Lisa and I were lucky to get a project EU-funded project that involved Carlo and Elizabeth, and another brilliant student of Carlo, the Austrian neuropsychologist, Margareta Hittmair (Delazer). Together we tested many neurological patients and were able to uncover the modular structure of the mathematical abilities in the adult brain – that is, the brain seems to be organized into separate components for each arithmetical operation, for recalling arithmetical facts, and for using arithmetical procedures, and for reading and for writing numbers.

Then I started wonder *why* the parietal lobe that was so critical – a question that hadn't been asked at that time. Then came another happy event. Another UCL colleague, Tim Shallice, who also worked in Italy at SISSA (Scuola Internazionale Superiore di Studi Avanzati) in Trieste, had money for a conference at SISSA, and suggested we organize one on mathematical cognition. We managed to invite anybody who was anybody in this field – developmental psychologists, cognitive psychologists, neuropsychologists, an animal psychologist and a philosopher, along with the only two scientists who were imaging the brain while doing mathematical tasks, plus, and this was critical, their students. Many of these people had never discussed mathematical cognition outside their narrow discipline, but now they had the perfect opportunity. This meeting gave rise to the two EU networks I mentioned, and these involved eight labs in six countries.

You will see many of their names in this book – Rochel Gelman, Karen Fuson, Randy Gallistel, Marcus Giaquinto, Mark Ashcraft, Stanislas Dehaene, Laurent Cohen, Xavier Seron, Karen Wynn, Jamie Campbell – and the students – Lisa, Margarete, Mauro Pesenti, Alessia Granà, Luisa Girelli, Marie-Pascale Noël, Etienne Koechlin, John Whalen, Anne Aubrun, Sven Blankenberger (Marco Zorzi, then a PhD student at SISSA, wasn't officially at the meeting, but would pop in from time to time) – and to them all I am immensely grateful. Carlo's students continued to join my lab and do their PhD with me. They have continued to contribute enormously to the development of the field – Manuela Piazza, Marinella Cappelletti, Teresa Iuculano, Raffaella Moro, Luisa Girelli. Through EU schemes I have been enormously lucky to work with Elena Rusconi, Andrea Mechelli, Slava Karolis, Petra Vetter, Fulvia Castelli, Sara Fabbri and Sara Caviola, Daniela Lucangeli, Pekka Räsänen, Alessia Granà, Marco Zorzi, Eva Spolaore and Silvia Pagano. My own work on the development of numerical abilities has been carried out with the great developmentalist, Bob Reeve, and his team at Melbourne University in Australia. In London, besides Tim and Elizabeth, I have been fortunate to collaborate with Michael Kopelman of St Thomas's Hospital and my colleagues Cathy Price, Vincent Walsh, Domenica Bueti, Roi Cohen Kadosh and Bahador Bahrami. My first study of dyscalculia was carried out with Karin Landerl who spent a year in my lab supported by the Austrian government and Anna Bevan, yet another brilliant student. (Good science depends much more on luck than you might think.)

Of course, fundamental to working on dyscalculia requires the help of great teachers of dyscalculia learners, and I have learned so much from Kelly Fullarton and Mandy Nayton in Perth, Australia, and from long-term collaborations with the late Dorian Yeo, Jane Emerson, and Trish Babtie, who kindly read through all the chapters and made important suggestions for improvements. My approach to intervention has been shaped, not only by these teachers, but crucially by my colleague and partner, Diana Laurillard.

I've also learned an enormous amount from the dyscalculics I have worked with over the years – many children and many adults. Some prefer to remain unnamed, or anonymized ("Charles", "Julie" and "Cathy"); but others are out and proud, including Paul Moorcraft (a book about dyscalculia), Alexa Raisbeck (an art installation) and Vivienne Parry (a radio programme).

I write in hope that dyscalculia becomes more widely recognized by educational authorities, and by teachers, parents and, not least, by its sufferers. I write in the hope that it becomes a required component of training teachers and educational psychologists.

References

Abeel, S. (2007). *My Thirteenth Winter: A Memoir.* New York: Scholastic.

Adlam, F. (2012). *Dyscalculia Matters: Effective Ways of Working with Children Who Struggle with Maths.* Essential Resources Ltd.

Attwood, T. *Dyscalculia Practice Activities.* First & Best in Education Ltd.

Babtie, P., & Emerson, J. (2015). *Understanding Dyscalculia and Numeracy Difficulties: A Guide for Parents, Teachers and Other Professionals.* London: Jessica Kingsley Publishers.

Bird, R. (2007). *The Dyscalculia Toolkit.* London: Paul Chapman Publishing.

Chinn, S. (2007). *Dealing with Dyscalculia: Sum Hope.* London: Souvenir Press Ltd.

Dowrick, N. (2015). Numbers count: a large-scale intervention for young children who struggle with mathematics. In R. Cohen Kadosh & A. Dowker (Eds), *Oxford Handbook of Numerical Cognition* (pp. 1099–1117). Oxford: OUP.

Emerson, J., & Babtie, P. (2013). *The Dyscalculia Assessment* (2nd ed.). London: Bloomsbury Education.

Emerson, J., & Babtie, P. (2014). *The Dyscalculia Solution: Teaching number sense.* London: Bloomsbury Education.

Henderson, A. (2012). *Dyslexia, Dyscalculia and Mathematics: A Practical Guide*, 2nd ed. Abingdon: Routledge.

Hornigold, J. (2015). *Dyscalculia Pocketbook.* Alresford: Teachers' Pocketbooks.

Moorcraft, P. (2014). *It Just Doesn't Add Up.* Croydon, Surrey: Filament Publishing Ltd.

Morton, J., & Frith, U. (1995). Causal modelling: a structural approach to developmental psychopathology. In D. Cichetti & D. Cohen (Eds), *Manual of Developmental Psychopathology* (Vol. 1, pp. 357–390). New York: John Wiley.

1

What is dyscalculia? It's not just being bad at maths

We all know that maths is an important life skill, even though many people are happy to admit that they are "crap at maths". By contrast, most people are not be prepared to say that they are bad at grammar, speaking or reading. In fact, poor maths is a more of a handicap in the workplace than poor literacy (Bynner & Parsons, 1997). Men and women with poor numeracy, have poorer educational prospects, earn less, and are more likely to be unemployed, in trouble with the law, and be sick (Parsons & Bynner, 2005).

The importance of mathematics instruction has been stressed, quite rightly, in many official reports in the UK, the US and other nations. Napoleon famously said that mathematics is "intimately connected with the prosperity of the state". In his foreword to the Cockcroft report on maths teaching in 1982, Sir Keith Joseph, Secretary of State for Education and Science, wrote, "Few subjects are as important to the future of the nation as mathematics" (Cockcroft, 1982). Since Cockcroft, in the UK alone there has been Professor Adrian Smith's report on post-14 maths (Smith, 2004), and Sir Peter Williams's report on primary maths (Williams, 2008). Similarly, the US National Research Council (National Research Council. Committee on Early Childhood Mathematics, 2009) noted that: "The new demands of international competition in the 21st century require a workforce that is competent in and comfortable with mathematics;" and to that end: "The committee [of experts] was charged with examining existing research in order to develop appropriate mathematics learning objectives for preschool children; providing evidence-based insights related to curriculum, instruction, and teacher education for achieving these learning objectives" (p. 1). In 2011, the OECD's report, *The High Cost of Low Educational Performance*, demonstrated that the standard of maths drives GDP growth: the standard in 1960 was a good predictor of economic growth up to 2000; and the improvement in educational standards from 1975 to 2000 was highly correlated with improvement in economic growth. In particular, the report looked at the potential effects of improving standards in maths. So, for example, they found that if the UK improved the standard of the 11% of children who failed to reach the PISA minimum level (which is not very high), to the minimum level, then the effect on GDP (Gross domestic product) growth would be about 0.44%. Not much you might think, but with an average rate of GDP growth of 1.5%, this would be a massive and cumulative increase of nearly one-third. The accountancy firm, KPMG, estimated the cost to the UK of poor maths in terms of lost direct and indirect taxes, unemployment benefits, justice costs, and additional educational costs, was £2.4 *billion* per year (Gross et al., 2009).

One cause of poor mathematical ability is developmental dyscalculia,[1] which is a handicap people are born with and which can persist into adulthood. In this way, it is comparable with dyslexia, which is also a condition someone is born with and persists into adulthood. I will deal with characteristics and causes of dyscalculia, as well as how to help in the following chapters. Unfortunately for dyscalculics, their teachers and their parents, dyscalculia does not have a high public profile. As the UK government's chief scientific adviser wrote: "Developmental dyscalculia is currently the poor relation of dyslexia, with a much lower public profile. But the consequences of dyscalculia are at least as severe as those for dyslexia" (Beddington et al., *Nature*, 2008, summarizing Government Office of Science report: *Mental Capital and Wellbeing*).

Terminology

It is not surprising that many people have become confused about dyscalculia. Here are some terms that are widely used. I list their principal official users, and also some of the scientists associated with each term. The pioneer Ladislav Kosc was the first to use the term *dyscalculia* to refer to a specific developmental condition. He defined it as follows:

> Developmental dyscalculia is a structural disorder of mathematical abilities which has its origin in a genetic or congenital disorder of those parts of the brain that are the direct anatomico-physiological substrate of the maturation of the mathematical abilities adequate to age, without a simultaneous disorder of general mental functions.
>
> (1970a, cited in 1974, p 47)

This is essentially the definition that I will use, modified in the light of subsequent research. It stresses its congenital and neurological basis, which many studies have neglected.

Kosc was careful to distinguish dyscalculia from just being bad at maths. He wrote:

> If a person has had inadequate instruction, or if a child because of neurosis, objective illness, or fatigue is not able to demonstrate his potential abilities or

---

1 Dyscalculia, like dyslexia, can be a condition you are born with, that is a developmental condition. It can also be acquired as a consequence of brain damage. I will use the term "dyscalculia" to mean the development type, unless specifically mentioned. See Chapter 7 on acquired dyscalculia.

directly acquired knowledge or skills adequately, this is not a *disorder* of these abilities as such but merely a deficit which is called … *pseudo-dyscalculia*.

(Kosc, 1974, p. 49)

- Dyscalculia or developmental dyscalculia (Kosc, US Department of Education, and many scientific papers, this book)
- Specific disorder of arithmetical skills (ICD 10, see below)
- Mathematics disorder (DSM IV, see below)
- Specific learning disorder with impairment in mathematics (DSM 5, see below)
- Mathematics/mathematical learning difficulty, MLD (Mazzocco, Geary, and many scientific papers).

So what is dyscalculia? Different authorities use different terminologies, and different criteria, and these official definitions, however vague, incoherent and unfounded, are nevertheless important from a practical point of view.

Dyscalculia is whatever your authorities think it is

Dyscalculia, or the local term for it, is whatever your authorities think it is. This may enable the parent, teacher, and sufferer, to request special help. This can be special help with exams, along the lines that dyslexics get help with exams in terms of extra time and the opportunity to use computers if handwriting is difficult. It can also mean help with learning. Again, dyslexics can get specialized teaching. There are places in the world where this approach can be useful, for example, Italy's Law 170 (see Box 1.1). This law provides for both recognition of the condition and help for overcoming its consequences.

Box 1.1 Italy's Law 170

Nuove norme in materia di disturbi specifici di apprendimento in ambito scolastico (New regulations concerning specific disorders of learning).

- Article 1.1. The present law recognizes dyslexia, dysgraphia, dysorthographia and dyscalculia as Specific Learning Disabilities.… They manifest themselves in cases of adequate cognitive capacities, and in absence of neurological or sensory deficits. Yet, they constitute an important limitation for daily activities.
- Article 1.5. The present law refers to dyscalculia as a specific deficit which manifests itself as a difficulty in grasping the automatisms of calculation and number processing.

(*continued overleaf*)

3

> ■ Article 2 states among other things, that there will be appropriate teaching to realize potential, a reduction in social and emotional consequence, train teachers appropriately, make people aware of the problem, promote early diagnosis and rehabilitation, and ensure equal opportunities to develop social and professional capacities.

The Individuals with Disabilities Education Act (IDEA) in USA recognizes dyscalculia (along with dyslexia). The Office of Special Education and Rehabilitative Services of the USA's Department of Education requires state and local education authorities to carry out appropriate assessments and to provide appropriate help.

> The Office of Special Education Programs (OSEP) funds a large network of technical assistance centers that develop materials and resources to support States, school districts, schools, and teachers to improve the provision of services to children with disabilities, including materials on the use of accommodations ... [which refers] to the various components of a free appropriate public education, including special education, related services, supplementary aids and services, and program modifications or supports for school personnel, as well as accommodations for students taking assessments.
>
> (Yudin, 2015)

The problem with this approach is that the authorities may not recognize dyscalculia; and even if they do, the authorities may not provide support, such as provision for additional money to buy in specialized help, or special provision ("accommodations") in the school.

Here is one example of failure to recognize from the UK Department for Education in 2016. It has dropped all the useful material about dyscalculia that had been there until 2015. However, a previous UK government did have *dyscalculia* on its website and in its publications. Here is the definition in *Guidance to support pupils with dyslexia and dyscalculia* published by the Department for Education and Skills in 2001:

> Dyscalculia is a condition that affects the ability to acquire arithmetical skills. Dyscalculic learners may have difficulty understanding simple number concepts, lack an intuitive grasp of numbers, and have problems learning number facts and procedures. Even if they produce a correct answer or use a correct method, they may do so mechanically and without confidence.... Purely dyscalculic learners who have difficulties only with number will have cognitive and language abilities in the normal range, and may excel in nonmathematical subjects.

First it describes the actual cognitive differences between the dyscalculic and typically developing peers, and not just that they may be slower and more limited in their acquisition of arithmetical skills. So it is not just that they are worse at arithmetic, which may have many causes. The dyscalculic disability is identified in terms of a particular cognitive deficit – a deficit in understanding simple number concepts and having an intuitive grasp of numbers.

Dyscalculia: it is what professionals think it is

Usually this will mean a special educational needs coordinator or an educational psychologist, but sometimes it can mean a medical doctor or a psychiatrist. These professionals may provide an assessment that recognizes dyscalculia, and indeed, can recommend the help that is needed. These professionals are important because the authorities do not specify what the assessments or the help should be. This is left to the professionals, and professionals will use definitions and criteria provided by professional organisations such as the American Psychiatric Association or the World Health Organisation.

Professional definitions

1. The Diagnostic and Statistical Manual of Mental Disorders, fourth Edition. DSM-IV

This is the "old testament" of categories of disorders devised by the American Psychiatric Association in the USA. It gives the following diagnostic criteria for "Mathematics Disorder" (Section 315.1)

A. Mathematical ability, as measured by individually administered standardized tests, is substantially below that expected given the person's chronological age, measured intelligence, and age-appropriate education.
B. The disturbance in Criterion A significantly interferes with academic achievement or activities of daily living that require mathematical ability.
C. If a sensory deficit is present, the difficulties in mathematical ability are in excess of those usually associated with it.

The first point to note is that the "standardized test" is not specified. If it is a standardized test of arithmetic, then there will be many reasons why a child may underperform, as we will see, especially in Chapter 3.

The second point to note is that this is a "discrepancy" criterion, which rules out by definition the possibility that someone can have both a mathematics disorder and low general cognitive ability; and it presumably implies that low measured intelligence is sufficient to cause the symptoms of "mathematics disorder". Indeed, for learners with equivalently poor performance on the standardized test, the one with the higher IQ is more likely to be granted the classification of Mathematics Disorder.

No justification is presented either for the terminology nor the evidential base for this classification. In fact, DSM-IV claims, again without evidence, that the prevalence of Mathematical Disorder is 1%. We will return to this in Chapter 2.

One practical problem is that it "operates a 'wait to fail' method, because it is unlikely that a significant discrepancy will be found" in the first two or three years of school This means delayed diagnosis, and delayed intervention. In fact, this definition can discourage intervention, because improvements achieved through sustained intervention may mean a reversal of diagnosis, and this in turn may lead to reduced support (*Understanding Learning Difficulties: A Practical Guide.* Dyslexia SPELD Foundation, Perth).

The second practical problem is that a discrepancy cannot be identified without a full, and often expensive, neuropsychological assessment of a wide range of cognitive capacities.

2. The Diagnostic and Statistical Manual of Mental Disorders, fifth Edition. DSM 5

The relevant section of the "new testament" is 315.1, under the heading *Learning disabilities* in the section on "neurodevelopmental disorders". It is a "Specific learning disorder with impairment in mathematics." The definition is quite different from DSM-IV.

A persistent difficulty learning academic skills for at least 6 months despite intervention targeting the area(s) of difficulty.

In number sense, fact and calculation, and in mathematical reasoning.
The academic and learning difficulties occur in the absence of:

1. Intellectual disabilities
2. Visual or hearing impairments
3. Mental disorders (e.g. depression, anxiety, etc.)
4. Neurological disorders
5. Psycho-social difficulty
6. Language differences
7. Lack of access to adequate instruction

The criterion for "persistent difficulty" is not defined, and the reason for 6 months failure to respond to intervention is not given. It is not clear what counts as an intellectual disability, nor a "neurological disorder". As we will see in Chapter 4, the brains of dyscalculics are different from those of non-dyscalculics. Does this difference count as a disorder? Although this does not immediately look like a discrepancy criterion, a poor showing on an IQ test could count as an intellectual disability, and hence rule out this maths-specific learning disability. Notice that the word dyscalculia is not used in DSM 5 (incidentally, neither is the word "dyslexia").

Why the change? "The DSM-5 Neurodevelopmental Work Group concluded that the many definitions of dyslexia and dyscalculia meant those terms would not be useful as disorder names or in the diagnostic criteria."

However, there are some virtues in the new definition. First, a full neuropsychological assessment may not be needed. Mandy Nayton, CEO of the Dyslexia SPELD Foundation in Perth, Australia, believes that it is easy to spot children dyscalculia in the first year of school because they fail to respond to the usual teaching methods. This means that intervention can start sooner than waiting for the child to fail.

3. The International Classification of Diseases Tenth Edition. ICD 10

This classification is produced by the World Health Organisation. ICD 10 is a more specific than the DSM criteria, but is it more helpful?

What constitutes "a billable ICD-10-CM code that can be used to indicate a diagnosis for reimbursement purposes?" (this, of course, is the US edition of ICD 10, where the carer or the individual has to request support from the insurer or from the state or local education authority). That is, what diagnosis will ensure that a child is entitled to special help for his or her mathematical difficulties? ICD 10 is the clearest and most specific of the widely-used classifications. In section F81.2 the term used is a "Specific disorder of arithmetical skills". This

> (i)nvolves a specific impairment in arithmetical skills that is not solely explicable on the basis of general mental retardation or of inadequate schooling. The deficit concerns mastery of basic computational skills of addition, subtraction, multiplication, and division rather than of the more abstract mathematical skills involved in algebra, trigonometry, geometry, or calculus.

Importantly, the disability is in arithmetic, not in other branches of mathematics. As we will see, a dyscalculic can be very bad at arithmetic, yet good at geometry, for example. However, there are problems.

Notice that the ICD definition excludes an impairment in arithmetical skills that is solely explicable on the basis of general mental retardation. That is, the child cannot be both stupid and have a specific disorder of arithmetical skills. Moreover, it excludes, in a later paragraph, "arithmetical difficulties associated with a reading or spelling disorder". Thus the child cannot be both dyscalculic and dyslexic. If they are dyslexic, they cannot be dyscalculic. For some unexplained reason, dyslexia takes precedence.

"Mental retardation" is another problem. Low measured IQ, or other tests of intelligence and general cognitive capacity, does not prevent high levels of mathematical skill. We know from the study of savants, with very low measured IQ or with other indicators of limited cognitive ability, that they can be superb calculators (Butterworth, 2006). We also know that IQ measures are poor predictors of mathematical competence, such that even individuals with very high measured IQ can be dyscalculic (Butterworth, Varma and Laurillard, 2011). This would mean that children with special educational needs would be excluded from a "billable code" because of their measured IQ. Now it may well be that these children can be drilled to perform moderately well on arithmetical problems, but the question addressed is much more interesting: do they have the conceptual basis and cognitive ability to develop their own valid strategies for calculation?

One further difficulty: ICD 10 excludes children poor on arithmetic due to "Inadequate schooling". Now ICD 10 does not define this term, so it is not possible to determine whether the child is classified as having a "Specific disorder of arithmetical skills" because of inadequate teaching. Teaching may be inadequate for a host of reasons. Here reading difficulties may well be relevant. If the classroom culture is heavily based on written language and the child has not overcome difficulties related to the use of this medium, then this could cause the child to fall behind in maths.

We will return to what adequate and appropriate teaching should be after we have identified what dyscalculia is.

A theory-based approach

At the root of the confusions about the criteria for dyscalculia, whichever term is used, and about the appropriate intervention, is the lack of theoretical perspective, and this is critical for understanding *why* a child fails to reach an expected level in maths.

Of course, what the expected level is will depend on social, economic, and importantly, political factors. One example is whether the educational authority – usually a government agency – recognizes dyscalculia as a "billable" category. It may fail to do so out of ignorance, since mathematical competence is a proxy for intelligence, or out of indolence if there is no parent pressure group to prod it into action. In the UK, and in many other countries, dyslexia is recognized precisely because there exist organizations that insist on its recognition. The authorities may not recognize dyscalculia because it could entail a commitment to provide support for those assessed as dyscalculia.

Without a theory, one is left with a criterion that could be set for economic or political reasons, or could simply be arbitrary: 35th percentile, for example, or the 16th, or 2nd percentiles. None of these criteria tells you what the learner needs. The problem is compounded when one considers different populations. Consider an international comparison, for example, the PISA 2012 study. The proportion of children below level 2 in the top 10 countries was around 10%, but in the worst performing countries it was between 60% and 75%. So what would count as dyscalculia in Singapore will be very different from what would count in Indonesia in terms of what the learner can and cannot do.

Here is the question that should be addressed: why is this child failing to understand what his or her classmates can understand? This is a theoretical question. In fact, it is the question that Kosc posed 40 years ago. He wanted to distinguish dyscalculia from pseudo-dyscalculia, which has quite different causes.

I will show that for about 5% of learners, the answer is that there is a deficit in very basic numerical concepts. That is, they will do poorly not only on tests that depend on the appropriateness of their schooling, or on social and economic status, and even home background, but also on tests that depend very little on these factors.

For example, these learners do poorly on test of the enumeration of small sets of objects, typically displays of dots. They will be slower and less accurate than their peers, and this is a stable measure of individual difference, and is a reliable predictor of the ease or difficulty of acquiring arithmetical competence (Reeve et al., 2012). They will also do poorly when asked to select the display with more dots, which also relies very little on education (Piazza et al., 2010). Why do these children do poorly on these very simple tests of number? Could it be that it is due to, what Kosc called, "a genetic or congenital disorder of those parts of the brain that are the direct anatomico-physiological substrate of the maturation of the mathematical abilities"?

Summary

- Different terms are used to refer to mathematical disabilities
  - Dyscalculia or developmental dyscalculia
  - Specific disorder of arithmetical skills
  - Mathematics disorder
  - Specific learning disorder with impairment in mathematics
  - Mathematics/mathematical learning difficulty
- These terms depend on different definitions and criteria and will not pick out exactly the same individuals.
- Local rules and regulations will determine which term and which criteria should be used. See Chapter 9 on assessment.
- I will use the term dyscalculia or developmental dyscalculia in this book, and will define it theoretically and empirically.

References

Butterworth, B. (2006). Mathematical expertise. In K. A. Ericsson, N. Charness, P. J. Feltovich, & R. R. Hoffmann (Eds), *Cambridge Handbook of Expertise and Expert Performance* (pp. 553–568). Cambridge: Cambridge University Press.

Butterworth, B., Varma, S., & Laurillard, D. (2011). Dyscalculia: From brain to education. *Science*, 332, 1049–1053. doi: 10.1126/science.1201536

Bynner, J., & Parsons, S. (1997). *Does Numeracy Matter?* London: Basic Skills Agency.

Cockcroft, W. H. (1982). *Mathematics Counts: Report of the Committee of Inquiry into the Teaching of Mathematics in Schools under the Chairmanship of Dr W H Cockcroft.* London: HMSO.

Gross, J., Hudson, C., & Price, D. (2009). *The Long Term Costs of Numeracy Difficulties.* Retrieved from: www.everychildachancetrust.org

Kosc, L. (1974). Developmental dyscalculia. *Journal of Learning Disabilities, 7,* 159–162.

Parsons, S., & Bynner, J. (2005). *Does Numeracy Matter More?* London: NRDC.

Piazza, M., Facoetti, A., Trussardi, A. N., Berteletti, I., Conte, S., Lucangeli, D., … Zorzi, M. (2010). Developmental trajectory of number acuity reveals a severe impairment in developmental dyscalculia. *Cognition, 116*(1), 33–41.

Reeve, R., Reynolds, F., Humberstone, J., & Butterworth, B. (2012). Stability and Change in Markers of Core Numerical Competencies. *Journal of Experimental Psychology: General, 141*(4), 649–666. doi: 10.1037/a0027520

Smith, A. (2004). *Making Mathematics Count: The Report of Professor Adrian Smith's Inquiry into Post-14 Mathematics Education.* Retrieved from: http://dera.ioe.ac.uk/4873/1/Maths InquiryFinalReport.pdf

Williams, P. (2008). *Independent Review of Mathematics Teaching in Early Years Settings and Primary Schools: Final Report.* (DCSF-00433–2008). Retrieved from: http://dera.ioe. ac.uk/8365/7/Williams%20Mathematics_Redacted.pdf

Yudin, M. K. (2015). Specific Learning Disabilities. Washington DC: United States Department of Education. Retrieved from www2.ed.gov/policy/speced/guid/idea/ memosdcltrs/guidance-on-dyslexia-10–2015.pdf

Number sense

Our intuitive understanding of numbers

LEVEL OF EXPLANATION	MEASURES		EDUCATIONAL CONTEXT
BEHAVIOURAL	**Number sense Chapter 2**		Society, school and home Chapter 8
COGNITIVE	Starter kit for learning arithmetic Chapter 3 Core deficit as the cause of dyscalculia Chapter 4		Assessment Chapter 9
	Development of arithmetic Chapter 5		Intervention Chapter 10
NEURAL	Brain structures and functions Chapter 6		Policy Chapter 11
	GENETIC AND OTHER CAUSES Chapter 7		

The infant's starter kit

When the infant first enters the world, the brain is not a "blank slate". The brain and the senses – vision, hearing, smell, taste and touch – are designed to make sense of the world, so that some features of the world are attended to and others, for the moment, ignored. The brain grows very rapidly after birth at a rate of 1% *per day* up to three months, and continues growing at 0.4% per day thereafter. In fact, brain volume doubles in 90 days from birth. There is also a very rapid increase in the volume of connections in this period. These changes are accompanied by very rapid changes in brain function – in the senses, in control of movement, and in cognition.

One obvious example of how we are not blank slates is colour vision. Humans, like many other creatures, come equipped with specialized neural mechanisms – the rods and cones in the retina of the eye and dedicated neural pathways to a specialized network in the brain – that enables them to identify and distinguish the colours in the environment. This, of course, is a very useful mechanism: it supports distinguishing ripe from unripe fruit, useful from useless flowers, friends from enemies, males from females (think ducks or peacocks). What is more, you cannot help seeing the world in colour. You may not pay attention to the colour of the object you saw, you may not remember its colour, but when you saw it, you saw it in colour. There is no switch to black and white. It is, what visual scientists call, a "primary visual property" of the world.

It has been proposed that seeing the world numerically is very much like seeing it in colour. The number of objects you see is a primary visual property of the world. You cannot help seeing the number of apples in the bowl. If the number is sufficiently small, you will identify that number – the "numerosity"

Box 2.1 Subitizing

Typical adult data that relates the number of dots on the horizontal axis with average time to give the correct number on the vertical axis (in milliseconds). There are two distinct slopes which are labelled "subitizing range" for up to four dots, and the "counting range" for more than four dots. The difference in the slopes suggests that there are two different and separate processes underlying this task. Subitizing (sometimes called "subitization") does not require serially enumerating the dots to arrive at the correct answer. You can immediately (subito) tell at a glance. For more than four dots, observers typically do serially enumerate, either verbally or unconsciously. Of course, it is possible to estimate without counting, and get the right answer. So in this range, observers may use a mix of estimating and counting. There is now extensive additional evidence, including evidence from neuroimaging, to support the two-process hypothesis.

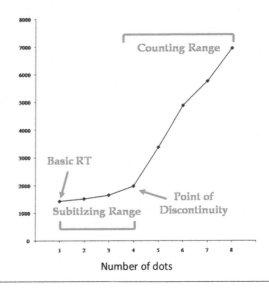

Number of dots

of the set of apples – accurately and immediately. That is what is termed "subitizing" (see Box 2.1). If the number is larger, you will have a rough sense of that number and you will be able to distinguish the numerosity of two sets of objects even if the sets are quite large and you don't know the exact numerosity of either. It is easy to tell whether there are more apples than oranges, if, for example there are 47 apples and 26 oranges, even if you don't know the exact number of apples and oranges, and even if they are mixed up.

Noticing that some things in the visual scene are objects, is clearly a precondition for enumerating them. From infancy (from the Latin *infans*, without speech) through toddlerhood to age four, the child's perceptual systems, especially vision, are becoming sharper, the faces and speech of individuals are recognized, language and social skills are being acquired, there is better control of actions, and inferences about the world are becoming increasingly sophisticated. How does arithmetic fit into this rapidly developing picture?

Number sense and the "number module"

It is useful to think of the learner as having a starter kit containing tools that can be brought to the task of learning arithmetic. The starter kit will contain tools for recognizing that an object is separate from the background and the surroundings, and that the object persists when not observed and even when it is wholly or partly hidden (Gibson & Spelke, 1983).

Now it may come as a surprise to know that one of the tools in the starter kit is specifically used for learning about numbers and arithmetic. The French neuroscientist, Stanislas Dehaene, a key figure in the study of human numerical abilities, has popularized the term "number sense" to refer to this innate ability.

What does it mean to say that we possess a "number module"? It means that learners enter the world with mental structures and principles that enables them to identify features of the world that are relevant to that domain and exclude those that are irrelevant, and this is done without formal or even informal instruction.

Another pioneer in this area, especially in relation to counting, is Rochel Gelman. Recently she listed what she called "core domains" that operate in an analogous modular way: "The … widely recognized core domains are those that govern the perception of and reasoning about objects, natural numbers, causality, the animate vs. inanimate, language, and sociality". (Gelman, 2015). Babies recognize smiling and will reciprocate smiles without being taught; they will notice when an object goes behind another object and will not be surprised when it reappears (contra the influential Swiss psychologist, Jean Piaget).

By contrast, non-core domains do require instruction, or self-instruction, and include things like playing chess, the piano or cricket, calculus, bread-making, computer programming, juggling, and so on and so on. These depend on culture and commitment to learning.

Infant's number sense

We know infants have number sense from studies of infant behaviour. Like adults, infants get bored with looking at the same thing over and over again, and get interested when something new is presented. Now the question is, will presenting the same number of objects, and especially, not the same objects, bore the infant? Will the infant stop looking at the display, and will the infant start looking longer if the *number* of objects changes? The answer is Yes. Of course, we have to be sure that it is the change of number that induces longer looking and not change of some other property of the display. According to Piaget, infants are still in the sensori-motor stage and unable to abstract away from the sensory properties of the display, so they should not be able to extract numerosities from displays since this would involve abstracting away from their visual properties – such as the amount of blackness (the dots are black against a white background), how densely packed the dots are, the total luminance, the amount of edge, and so on. In Figure 2.1, you can see an example of this. This is the display from the very first attempt to demonstrate an infant's response to change of number; Figure 2.2 shows a later study using larger numerosities.

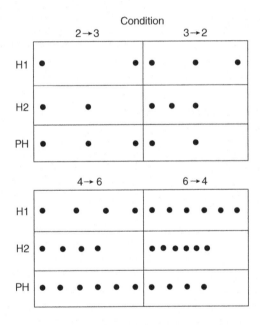

Figure 2.1 This was the first study to test whether infants of 22 weeks would notice when the number of objects in the display changed. The infant would see a habituation display H1 and H2 repeated until there was a 50% decrease in looking time averaged over three successive trials. Then there was a post habituation (PH) test using the same criterion. The results showed the infants look longer in PH for two dots changing to three, and three to two, but not six to four, or four to six (Starkey & Cooper, 1980).

Habituation

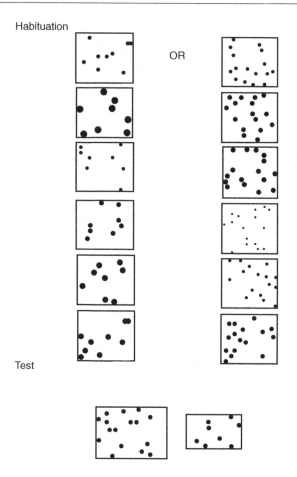

OR

Test

Figure 2.2 Do six-month-olds look longer when the number of dots changes? Another way of asking this: do infants habituate to a numerosity (number of dots) if it
is repeated several times, even though the display will look different each time? If
they do, then they should dishabituate – look longer – when a new numerosity – the
test – appears.

Results: Infants look longer at 8 vs 16, but not 8 vs 12.

Implication: Infants cannot be using non-numerical dimensions (such as the amount of
blackness because this changes with each display); but can make discriminations on the
basis of numerosity if the ratio between the habituation and test displays is large enough,
here 2:1, but not 3:2 (Xu & Spelke, 2000).

Infants will respond to changes of number, even if the objects are moving along
random trajectories, so the infants cannot have been responding to a change in
the pattern, since each of the rectangles was in constant motion, so they must
have extracted the numerosity from the moving displays (Van Loosbroek &
Smitsman, 1990).

These infants were relatively old – five months to eight months – but it is possible to show sensitivity to numerosity even in the first week of life (Antell & Keating, 1983). Indeed, it has been shown that infants in the first two days of life have a kind of abstract concept of numerosity that goes beyond just visual perception: they prefer – that is, they look longer at – a visual display that matches in *number* a sequence of tones they have just heard.

Is there an upper limit to the infant's concept of numerosity? Can she enumerate four, 10, or 100? Three seems to be the maximum, though infants in the Starkey & Cooper (1980) study distinguished four from three, but four for them may have represented just "more than three". On the other hand, infants are able not only to recognise small numerosities up to about four, they can distinguish larger numerosities provided the difference between them is big enough. So, infants can discriminate eight dots from 16 but not eight dots from 12 dots, as in Figure 2.2 (Xu & Spelke, 2000).

This infant ability – which, incidentally, is shared with many other creatures – is potentially a tool in the starter kit. Of course, to learn arithmetic other tools are needed, but these are not used only for learning arithmetic but deployed in a wide variety of tasks in a wide range of domains. These are usually called "domain-general" cognitive tools, that is, tools that can be applied to a wide range of different tasks. These will include intelligence, reasoning abilities, working memory, long-term memory, and attention. I also include language in this category. If the learner cannot understand what the teacher or carer says, or what's written in books of mathematics, it could be a tremendous handicap in learning arithmetic (see Chapter 3).

These contrast with "domain-specific" cognitive tools that apply solely to number and arithmetic.

Measuring the capacity of the number module

Numerosity discrimination

One widely used method is to determine how well an individual can discriminate numerosities by selecting the larger (or the smaller) numerosity. In Figure 2.3 I show the kind of stimuli that have been used to test this. The idea here is that the discrimination task taps the *Approximate Number System* which, as the name says, represents the numerosity of a set of objects only approximately. This is particularly relevant for sets greater than about four, since the smaller sets can be accurately and rapidly enumerated using a different mechanism, sometimes referred to as *subitizing*.

There are two ways of measuring the ability to do this. The first depends on how reliably an individual can pick the larger set. This gets harder, the more similar the numerosities are. In Figure 2.3, I give some examples. You can see for yourself that 2.3a is easier than 2.3b. This is sometimes called the "distance

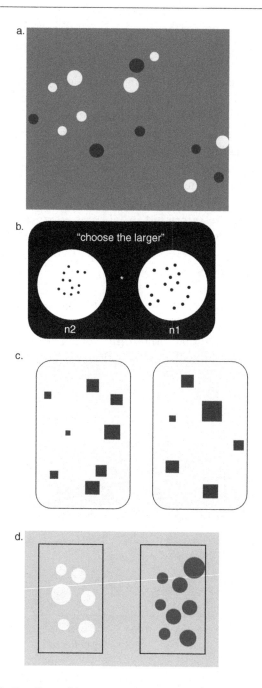

Figure 2.3 Types of stimuli used in numerosity discrimination tasks. **a.** Test: Are there more blue or more yellow dots? (Halberda et al., 2008). **b.** Test: Choose the panel with more dots. (Piazza et al., 2010). **c.** Test: Which side has more squares? (Iuculano et al., 2008). **d.** Which side has more dots? (Libertus et al., 2011).

effect"; that is, the greater the distance, or difference, between the two sets the easier the task, and the more likely you are to get it right. Now distance is sometimes presented as the absolute difference between the two sets – two in 2.3a but four in 2.3b. More usually it is given in terms of the *proportional difference* between the two sets. This follows one of the oldest laws in psychology, first identified by the German doctor and psychologist, Ernst Weber (1795–1878). Weber tested this using weight, but all kinds of stimuli – brightness, loudness, and pitch – follow the same law.

The exact value of the proportional difference that an individual can reliably discriminate will depend on the stimulus dimension – loudness is easier than brightness – and the sensitivity of the individual. It is the *sensitivity of the individual* that we are interested in when assessing skill at discriminating numerosities: that is, Mr A is more sensitive than Mr B, because he can reliably discriminate a 10% difference while Mr B can only reliably discriminate when the difference is 20%. Sensitivity is sometimes called the Weber Fraction, after Ernst Weber.

Figure 2.4 shows the result of the first study to relate arithmetical ability to sensitivity, by Halberda and colleagues.

Now it is easy to see that, other things being equal, the set with more objects will also have more blue (2.3a, c), or more black (2.3b), so how can we be sure

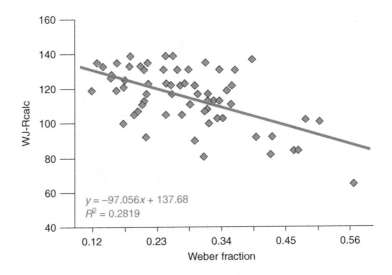

Figure 2.4 The relationship between the Weber fraction of individual students and their performance on a standardized test of arithmetic – WJ-Rcalc (Woodcock-Johnson Psycho-Educational Battery Revised calculation subtest). R^2 is a way of measuring the effect of the Weber fraction on the arithmetic test; a value of 0.28 means that there is moderate but significant effect, but that other factors are also important.

that the observer is making a decision on the basis of the amount of blue or the amount of black rather than the number of dots? Indeed, numerosity discrimination is biased by total dot area (Gebuis & Reynvoet, 2012a; 2012b). Several methods have been tried. The total area of blue or black in the two sets can be equated; but then the larger set will have smaller dots on average, so that observers may be making a judgment on the basis of dot size: picking the set with smaller dots will mean picking the set with more dots. Or dot size can be held constant – in which case, of course, total area will be a clue to the larger set. In at least one study, half the trials used equated area and the other half of the trials used constant dot size (Libertus et al., 2011). Another method, which I think is preferable, is to vary total area and dot size randomly, as was done with stimuli in 2.2c, so that the panel with greater number of squares also had the greatest total area of blue one third of the time; for another third, the panel with the greater number had the same total area as the panel with fewer squares; and one-third of the time the panel with the greater number had less total area of blue (Iuculano et al., 2008).

Box 2.2 The analogue magnitude system

Mathematicians have for centuries used space as a model for numbers, and this has transformed how humans have thought about number. To take one very simple example, putting numbers on a line beginning with zero on the left, probably encouraged mathematicians to wonder what sort of numbers were to the left of the zero. Hence, we had the very useful idea of negative numbers. Then there is the idea of locating points in a coordinate space using positive and negative numbers (Cartesian coordinates). More generally, mathematicians like to integrate numbers and spatial representations. The question is under what conditions the brain of a human non-mathematician does the same thing. In 1993, Stanislas Dehaene, a French mathematician and neuroscientist, published two papers suggesting that this is exactly what the human brain does.

In one paper, he showed that human adults have a preference for small numbers (<5) being on the left of space and large numbers (6–9) on the right. He asked his participants to decide whether a number was odd or even by pressing a left key or a right key. If the number was small, they would be faster with the left key, and if it was large they were faster than the right key. This foundational experiment has led to hundreds of replications and a few failures to replicate. This result has been interpreted revealing a "mental number line" in the head, a kind of vector with both magnitude and direction (left to right) (Dehaene et al., 1993).

(continued overleaf)

Dehaene's second paper in 1993, with neuroscientist Jean-Pierre Changeux, created a computer model of numerical development and processing. In this, they showed how the number line might arise without an organism knowing any of the familiar symbols (Dehaene & Changeux, 1993). This meant that idea of the numerosity of a set of objects could be extracted from the environment by any organism with requisite computing power, including non-human organisms. They also specified the number line in more detail. Each number was represented by a distribution of activation on the line, with the peak of the distribution around the number. Another way of thinking about this is in terms of the probability of where a given numerosity will fall on the number line. Now, notice in the figure below that the representations of the numbers overlap. The distance between the numbers gives the "distance effect" – the representations of distant numbers will overlap less, so that it will be easier to select the larger, and quicker. Dehaene and Changeux introduced another modification: the number line is compressed (for example, logarithmically compressed). This, they felt, would be more consistent with how the individual neurons in the brain behave. It also provided a (slightly) better mathematical match for the distance effect.

Now, if the neural representation of numbers overlap, and is intrinsically probabilistic, then these representations are different from our familiar whole numbers. There is a step–change from 4 to 5, for instance. This has led many to refer to this kind of representation as "the approximate number system", which means that number are represented only approximately, rather than exactly, which is how we normally think of the whole numbers (integers).

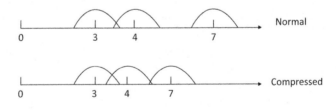

Numerosity enumeration

Another widely-used method for measuring individual numerosity-processing is simply asking the learner to name the number of objects in a display. Again, we can use two metrics: accuracy and speed. You can try this for yourself with the displays in Figure 2.5. Start with the leftmost panel. Try to be as fast and as accurate as possible.

Figure 2.5 These are the kinds of stimuli used in dot enumeration tasks. Try naming the numbers starting with the leftmost panel.

Number sense and arithmetic

One way of discovering whether number sense is a critical foundation for learning arithmetic is see if your ability to carry out number sense tasks such as the ones listed above, is related to your ability to learn arithmetic. Of course, many other factors will be important in learning arithmetic – including the quality of formal teaching and exposure to numbers in the home. I deal with these factors in detail in Chapter 8. First, we will look at individual differences in number sense and their relationship with arithmetical ability.

Numerosity discrimination

This kind of study was pioneered by three US psychologists, Justin Halberda, Lisa Feigenson, and Michèle Mazzocco from Johns Hopkins University in Baltimore. They documented individual differences in the sensitivity of learners aged 14, and related their ability to discriminate numerosities with stimuli like 2.1a, with detailed records of their performance on standardized arithmetic tests from kindergarten onwards (Halberda et al., 2008). They found a significant relationship between the ability to discriminate and measures of arithmetic at all ages. This finding has been supported by studies of pre-schoolers (Gilmore et al., 2007) and by studies of children in their first year of school (Gilmore et al., 2010); and by a recent very large-scale web-based study across the age-range (Halberda et al., 2012).

Now you might imagine that this basic capacity would be more relevant when you are just starting out to learn arithmetic than when you have become skilled, and indeed some lab-based (as opposed to web-based) studies do show a relationship for children but not for adults (e.g. Inglis et al., 2011). In fact, some studies fail to show a relationship even in children (Holloway & Ansari, 2009; Iuculano et al., 2008).

Numerosity identification

The usual way to measure individual differences in number sense is to ask participants to name the number of dots in a display like Figure 2.5. This is usually termed *dot enumeration*, and the critical measure here is the time taken to correctly name the number of dots. This measure can then be related to differences to a measure of arithmetical competence.

We carried out a longitudinal study using dot enumeration in Melbourne, Australia, led by Bob Reeve, an eminent developmental psychologist (Reeve et al., 2012). This was a *prospective* study; that is, it tested children in kindergarten, and then followed them for the next five years to see if number sense in kindergarten predicted arithmetical competence at subsequent occasions. Since this is the most complete longitudinal study of this issue, I will describe it in some detail. One hundred and fifty-nine children were tested seven times until the age of 11, including tests of dot enumeration on five separate occasions at 6 years, 7 years, 8.5 years, 9 years and 11 years. As well as dot enumeration, we tested non-verbal intelligence (Ravens Coloured Progressive Matrices) and the ability to select the larger of two digits – e.g. 2 or 8 – which is another standard test. The measures of arithmetical competence were appropriate for age and curriculum: at age six, it was single-digit addition; at nine and a half, two digit addition, subtraction, and multiplication, and at age ten, three digit subtraction, multiplication and division.

We discovered that the children in kindergarten, and indeed on subsequent testing fell into three distinct groups based on their dot enumeration performance, and tended to stay in these groups throughout the study. We labelled the groups Slow, Medium and Fast. Although all children got faster at the task as they got older, as you would expect, each child's speed relative to their peers stayed the same. That is, children in the Slow group were always slower than children in the other two groups at each age we tested them.

We found that group membership in kindergarten predicted age-appropriate arithmetical performance up to the age of 11 (see Figure 2.6). These findings are very strong evidence that arithmetic builds on this inherited domain-specific capacity, and suggests that tests in kindergarten can identify children who are at risk of difficulty in learning arithmetic.

The number line task

This task is a quick educational tool to see if a learner still understood the meaning of number words and number symbols (Bright et al., 1988). It has also been used for a long time with patients brain damage as a quick test of their number understanding (Cohen et al., 2000; van Harskamp et al., 2002). Here is how it works: We draw a line on paper with the left end defined as 0 and the right end defined as 100, for example, and ask that the patient or learner to mark 76, say, on that line (the patient studies typically use a "thermometer" orientation with 0 or 1 at the bottom and 100 or 1000 at the top). How well numbers are understood is estimated by how accurate the mark is. This simple test is now part of a standardized battery for assessing adult numerical abilities (Semenza et al., 2014).

Several studies have found that accuracy on this task correlates with arithmetical ability in children (Booth & Siegler, 2008; Siegler & Opfer, 2003), especially when one takes account of improvements in accuracy as the child gets older (Reeve et al., 2015). See Figure 2.7.

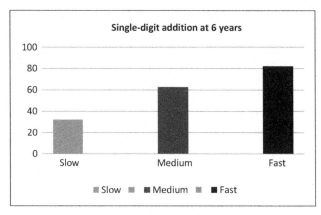

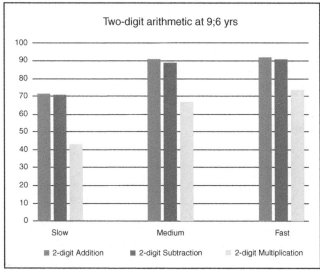

Figure 2.6 This shows age-appropriate arithmetical performance of group of 159 children we tested from kindergarten to age 11 years. We gave these children a dot enumeration task where the child had to name the number of dots (up to nine dots) as quickly as possible. A statistical technique called "cluster analysis" identified three clusters based on their speed and accuracy, which we called Slow, Medium and Fast. Seven percent of the children fell into the Slow cluster. As you can see, the Slow cluster were always worse than the other two groups at each testing age. We suggest that a simple dot enumeration task at the beginning of formal school is a good way of identifying children at risk of falling behind in arithmetic (Reeve et al., 2012). (*continued overleaf*)

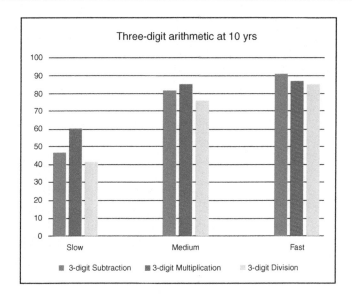

Figure 2.6 (*Continued*)

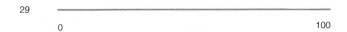

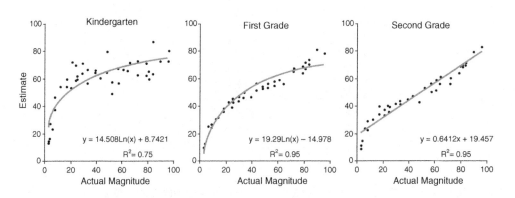

Figure 2.7 The top panel shows an example of the task the children undertook. They had to mark where they thought 29 should be on the line below. They marked 24 numbers altogether on separate lines. The bottom panel shows the responses of children at different ages. As they got older they became more accurate (Siegler & Booth, 2004). In a subsequent study they found that accuracy correlated significantly with performance on a standardized arithmetic test (Booth & Siegler, 2008).

At the same time, other studies have failed to find an association (Iuculano et al., 2008). Siegler and colleagues, among others, have claimed that the number line task reflects a "mental number line" that is oriented left to right, and that it is innately logarithmic. This would explain the shape of the Kindergarten and First Grade curves in Figure 2.7, which show a logarithmic relationship between the target and the estimate. Learning that numbers are in fact equally spaced – that is, linear not log – straightens out the mental number line.

However, it has been shown the task is just as easy with the right end defined as 0 and the left defined as 100 (Iuculano & Butterworth, 2011; Karolis et al., 2011). Nevertheless, longitudinal change in number line task accuracy is useful predictor of maths ability (Reeve et al., 2015).

Summary

- There is an innate number sense system, which is a component of what I have termed the "number module"
- Individual differences in number sense ability correlates with arithmetical ability
- The fact that it can be measured using different methods giving largely comparable results suggests that number sense is a valid construct

These findings set the scene for the central claim in this book: dyscalculia is a deficit in the number module. We can use tests like the ones above, and in particular dot enumeration, as a way of identifying learners – children and adults – who have a deficit in the key tool in the starter kit.

References

Antell, S. E., & Keating, D. P. (1983). Perception of numerical invariance in neonates. *Child Development*, 54, 695–701.

Booth, J. L., & Siegler, R. S. (2008). Numerical Magnitude Representations Influence Arithmetic Learning. *Child Development*, 79(4), 1016–1031. doi: 10.1111/j.1467–8624.2008.01173.x

Bright, G. W., Behr, M. J., Post, T. R., & Wachsmuth, I. (1988). Identifying fractions on number lines. *Journal for Research in Mathematics Education*, 19(3), 215–232.

Cohen, L., Dehaene, S., Chochon, F., Lehericy, S., & Naccache, L. (2000). Language and calculation within the parietal lobe: a combined cognitive, anatomical and fMRI study. *Neuropsychologia*, 38, 1426–1440.

Dehaene, S., & Changeux, J.-P. (1993). Development of elementary numerical abilities: A neuronal model. *Journal of Cognitive Neuroscience*, 5, 390–407.

Dehaene, S., Bossini, S., & Giraux, P. (1993). The mental representation of parity and numerical magnitude. *Journal of Experimental Psychology: General*, 122, 371–396.

Gebuis, T., & Reynvoet, B. (2012a). The interplay between nonsymbolic number and its continuous visual properties. *Journal of Experimental Psychology: General*, 141(4), 642–648. doi: 10.1037/a0026218

Gebuis, T., & Reynvoet, B. (2012b). The Role of Visual Information in Numerosity Estimation. *PLoS ONE*, 7(5), e37426. doi: 10.1371/journal.pone.0037426

Gelman, R. (2015). Learning in core and non-core number domains. *Developmental Review*, 38, 185–200. doi: 10.1016/j.dr.2015.07.010

Gibson, E. J., & Spelke, E. S. (1983). The development of perception. In J. H. Flavell & E. M. Markman (Eds), *Handbook of child psychology*: Vol. 3. Cognitive development 4th ed (pp. 1–76). New York: Wiley.

Gilmore, C. K., McCarthy, S. E., & Spelke, E. S. (2007). Symbolic arithmetic knowledge without instruction. *Nature* (447), 589–592.

Gilmore, C. K., McCarthy, S. E., & Spelke, E. S. (2010). Non-symbolic arithmetic abilities and mathematics achievement in the first year of formal schooling. *Cognition*, 115(3), 394–406.

Halberda, J., Mazzocco, M. M. M., & Feigenson, L. (2008). Individual differences in non-verbal number acuity correlate with maths achievement. *Nature*, 455, 665–668 doi: 10.1038/nature07246

Halberda, J., Ly, R., Wilmer, J. B., Naiman, D. Q., & Germine, L. (2012). Number sense across the lifespan as revealed by a massive Internet-based sample. *Proceedings of the National Academy of Sciences*, 109(28), 11116–11120. doi: 10.1073/pnas.1200196109

Holloway, I. D., & Ansari, D. (2009). Mapping numerical magnitudes onto symbols: The numerical distance effect and individual differences in children's mathematics achievement. *Journal of Experimental Child Psychology*, 103(1), 17–29.

Inglis, M., Attridge, N., Batchelor, S., & Gilmore, C. (2011). Non-verbal number acuity correlates with symbolic mathematics achievement: But only in children. *Psychonomic Bulletin & Review*, 18(6), 1222–1229. doi: 10.3758/s13423-011-0154-1

Iuculano, T., & Butterworth, B. (2011). Understanding the real value of fractions and decimals. *Quarterly Journal of Experimental Psychology*, 64 ((11)), 2088–2098. doi: 10.1080/17470218.2011.604785

Iuculano, T., Tang, J., Hall, C., & Butterworth, B. (2008). Core information processing deficits in developmental dyscalculia and low numeracy. *Developmental Science*, 11(5), 669–680.

Karolis, V., Iuculano, T., & Butterworth, B. (2011). Mapping numerical magnitudes along the right lines: Differentiating between scale and bias. *Journal of Experimental Psychology: General*, 140(4), 693–706. doi: 10.1037/a0024255

Libertus, M. E., Feigenson, L., & Halberda, J. (2011). Preschool acuity of the approximate number system correlates with school math ability. *Developmental Science*, 14, 1292–1300. doi: 10.1111/j.1467-7687.2011.01080.x

Piazza, M., Facoetti, A., Trussardi, A. N., Berteletti, I., Conte, S., Lucangeli, D., Dehaene, S., Zorzi, M. (2010). Developmental trajectory of number acuity reveals a severe impairment in developmental dyscalculia. *Cognition*, 116(1), 33–41.

Reeve, R., Paul, J. M., & Butterworth, B. (2015). Longitudinal changes in young children's 0–100 to 0–1000 number-line error signatures. *Frontiers in Psychology*, 6, 647. doi: 10.3389/fpsyg.2015.00647

Reeve, R., Reynolds, F., Humberstone, J., & Butterworth, B. (2012). Stability and Change in Markers of Core Numerical Competencies. *Journal of Experimental Psychology: General*, 141(4), 649–666. doi: 10.1037/a0027520

Semenza, C., Meneghello, F., Arcara, G., Burgio, F., Gnoato, F., Facchini, S., . . . Butterworth, B. (2014). A new clinical tool for assessing numerical abilities in neurological diseases: Numerical Activities of Daily Living. *Frontiers in Aging Neuroscience*, 6. doi: 10.3389/fnagi.2014.00112

Siegler, R. S., & Booth, J. L. (2004). Development of numerical estimation in young children. *Child Development*, 75(2), 428–444.

Siegler, R. S., & Opfer, J. E. (2003). The development of numerical estimation: Evidence for multiple representations of numerical quantity. *Psychological Science*, 14, 237–243.

Starkey, P., & Cooper, R. G., Jr. (1980). Perception of numbers by human infants. *Science*, 210, 1033–1035.

van Harskamp, N. J., Rudge, P., & Cipolotti, L. (2002). Are multiplication facts implemented by the left supramarginal and angular gyri? *Neuropsychologia*, 40, 1789–1793.

Van Loosbroek, E., & Smitsman, A. W. (1990). Visual perception of numerosity in infancy. *Developmental Psychology*, 26, 916–922.

Xu, F., & Spelke, E. (2000). Large number discrimination in 6-month-old infants. *Cognition*, 74, B1–B11.

3

The arithmetic starter kit

LEVEL OF EXPLANATION	MEASURES	EDUCATIONAL CONTEXT
BEHAVIOURAL	Number sense Chapter 2	Society, school and home Chapter 8
COGNITIVE	**Starter kit for learning arithmetic Chapter 3** Core deficit as the cause of dyscalculia Chapter 4	Assessment Chapter 9
	Development of arithmetic Chapter 5	Intervention Chapter 10
NEURAL	Brain structures and functions Chapter 6	Policy Chapter 11
	GENETIC AND OTHER CAUSES Chapter 7	

At the end of Chapter 2, I floated the idea that a good way of thinking about learning arithmetic is in terms of a cognitive "starter kit" containing tools essential for the job. In this chapter, I set out to explain the role of these tools.

The tools can be divided into two types:

■ "Domain-specific": the number module. This is the cognitive tool specific to numbers and arithmetic. In Chapter 2, I focused on *number sense* (or what I prefer to call *number abstraction*) – the way we extract or abstract numerical information from the environment – and showed that the individual differences in the ability to do this correlates with how well formal arithmetic is acquired. However, I didn't explain why this should be the case, except in a very general way. In this chapter, I will show that number abstraction is a component of a more complex capacity that I have called the "number module", which contains capacities for understanding *sets and their properties*, that enable the learner to *reason* about numbers.

■ "Domain-general" – these are cognitive capacities that the child applies to a wide range of tasks and to learning all curriculum subjects. These include reasoning abilities (often measured by IQ tests), working memory, long-term memory and attention. I also include language in this category. If the learner cannot understand what the teacher or carer says, or what's written in school textbooks, it could be a tremendous handicap in learning arithmetic.

Now, both types of tool – domain-general and domain-specific – are in the learner's starter kit, and both are needed to develop arithmetical competence, but, I will argue, it is the deficit in the domain-specific tool – what I have called the "number module" – that leads to dyscalculia. *The pattern of disabilities due to a defective number module is quite different from the disabilities caused by disabilities with domain-general tools.* I will deal with the effects of impairments in domain-general tools in Chapter 5, and I will show that they lead to quite distinct patterns of difficulties for the learner.

Domain-specific tools

The human being comes into the world *not* as a "blank slate" able to learn all things equally well using a generalized learning mechanism (Pinker, 2008). Rather, the human infant is born with specialized capacities – the modules – that make some things much easier to learn than others. The most widely-cited and celebrated is the ability to learn language. Most languages are horribly complex as anyone trying to learn another language as an adult can attest, with tricky rules and exceptions to rules, and vocabularies of 50,000 words or more. Yet babies pick up their native language apparently effortlessly without systematic formal instruction. According to Chomsky, this is because we are born with a language module: that is, language learners enter the world with mental structures and principles that enables them to identify features of the world that are relevant to the domain of language and exclude those that are irrelevant (Hauser et al., 2002; Pinker, 1994).

Another example of domain-specificity is seeing the world in colour. Again, we are born with the neural equipment for doing this, a complex network that runs from the rods and cones in the retina, via a series of neural relays to a specialized region of the brain. It works entirely automatically: we cannot help but see the world in colour. You cannot choose to see the world in black and white.

Is the same true for seeing the numbers of objects? According to David Burr and John Ross, two Australian visual scientists, the answer is yes (Burr & Ross, 2008). They argue that it is. That is, we cannot help but see the world numerically just as we cannot help but see the world in colour. We, and other creatures, can see that there are more fruit on this tree than that, that there are more enemies than friends (so we should flee and not fight). We and other creatures can calculate the rate of events in the environment, which means we can enumerate the number of events and divide this number into a measure of duration.

The idea that we humans are born with core knowledge of numbers and arithmetic is due originally to the American psychologists, Rochel Gelman and Charles Gallistel in their ground-breaking 1978 book *The Child's Understanding of Number*. In this account, infants were born with a number module that enabled them to identify small numerosities.

This book was a challenge to the very influential Swiss psychologist, Jean Piaget. He believed that the concept of number – of numerosity – was the result of the application of general reasoning abilities – domain-general tools – in interaction with the environment. For more on Piaget's position, see Chapter 5.

What does the number module do?

As we saw in Chapter 2, one of its functions is to extract numerical information from the environment. It does this automatically, just like extracting colour information from the environment. You do not have to will it, and you do not need to intend to do it, and, in fact, you cannot turn it off. This is the "number sense" function. This allows us to match and discriminate the numerosities present to our senses, usually vision, but could be auditory or tactile (Anobile et al., 2015).

It turns out that there is a very simple mechanism that could do this. Now I have suggested that number abstraction ability is innate. I take my lead from pioneering research on animal numerical abilities (Meck & Church, 1983). The central idea here is that our brain – and the brains of many, perhaps most, other creatures – contains a mechanism for enumerating experiences called an "accumulator". One way to think about it is as a click-counter (see Figure 3.1).

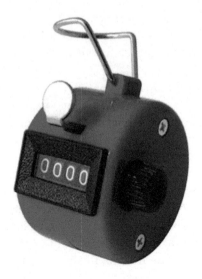

Figure 3.1 Click-counter: a very simple accumulator.

This is a very simple (and cheap) device requiring one key press for each item counted. It could readily be implemented in a small number of brain cells, so that even an insect with just one million brain cells would be able to count, as indeed has been demonstrated in bees and even in ants (Skorupski et al., 2018). Bigger brains are needed to decide what objects to count and categorize experiences into those to be counted and those to be ignored. So, for example, to count the number of squares in a display irrespective of whether the square is small or large or whether it's black or white, each square will be counted in the same way as one *unit*. Now the click-counter has a digital read out, but we cannot assume that the brain has the same. To cut a rather long story short, the neural accumulator represents a continuous quantity, rather like the level of liquid in a jug, but a jug which has calibration marks are on the side. The level of liquid will never be exactly on the calibration mark, but near enough and reliably enough, to represent numerosities. To persist with this metaphor, we can think of the units as being cupfuls of liquid being poured into the jug, one cupful per object counted (see Figure 3.2).

The accumulator mechanism needs just three very simple components:

1. A unit – the simplest and most basic *numerosity*. In Figure 3.2 the cup representing the unit of energy transferred into the accumulator
2. Adding – this is achieved by increasing the level of the accumulator by the fixed quantity
3. Calibration of the accumulator so that each level corresponds to a particular *numerosity*. This is important because the brain is inherently noisy so that a given level will vary a bit, and calibration will find the best fit for each numerosity.

It turns out that calibrating is important for linking levels in the accumulator with counting words (see Chapter 5).

Notice that the accumulator is entirely independent of what is counted, as long as the organism can categorise its experiences – visual, auditory, or whatever – into objects to be counted and those to be ignored. Gelman and Gallistel call this ability "number abstraction" since its function is to extract and abstractly represent the numerosity of sets: that is, the number of fingers on my hand has the same (abstract) number or numerosity as the number of chimes when Big Ben strikes five o'clock. The fives share no perceptual features – fingers are seen and felt, the chimes are heard: all they have in common is their fiveness.

According to their pioneering investigations, the module also contains what they call "domain-relevant structures". These are principles that help the child notice and use numerical information in their environment, such as seeing that there are more apples than oranges, and understanding that by putting a set of three smarties with a set of two smarties you get more smarties. Initially, these principles are not well-articulated, or even conscious, but they start the child on "right developmental path" (Gelman & Gallistel, 1978).

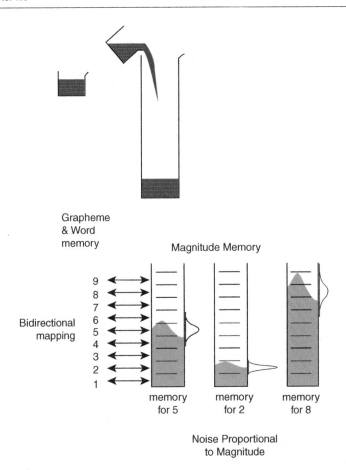

Figure 3.2 Accumulator counting: a metaphor. The cup represents a unit to be counted; the level of liquid in the accumulator represents the number of units counted, and the calibration indicates the numerosity, two, counted so far. Each count is stored in a memory. Here is shown the levels in memory, for five, two and eight. In learning to count with counting words or numerals (graphemes), the child has to learn to map between levels in the memories and words and the numerals. The brain is noisy, with noise proportional to magnitude, so this mapping will be the best estimate of the relevant level.

Adapted from Cordes et al., 2001; Leslie et al., 2008.

Infant's number abstraction

Gelman and Gallistel distinguish "number abstraction" from "number reasoning". Number abstraction is precisely that cognitive capacity that enables us – and many other animals – to identify, match and discriminate the numerosities of sets of objects when the sensory properties of the objects in the sets are different.

In fact, we know that infants can even match sets across the modalities of seeing and hearing where the objects have no sensory properties in common. For example, they can match the number of speakers they hear with the number of speakers they see: if they hear three speakers they will look longer at a display with three heads speaking than two heads speaking (Jordan & Brannon, 2006). This cross-modal matching, evident even in the first few hours of life (Izard et al., 2009), suggests that the number abstraction component of the number module is able to treat the numerosity of sets abstractly – that is, independently of their particular sensory properties.

This is important for arithmetical development because arithmetic is based on sets; and the property of sets I have called numerosity. Notice that sets are abstract – you can see or hear the members of the set – but you cannot see or hear the set. The numerosity property of the set is also abstract – an abstraction of an abstraction. This is why you can tell whether the number of fingers on your hand is the same (or different) from the number of chimes of Big Ben. To do this is an example of *number reasoning*, which goes beyond number abstraction but it depends on it. That is, the ability to determine whether two sets have the same or different numbers of objects is fundamental to learning arithmetic.

Now, not everyone agrees that infants have the capacity to represent sets and their properties. Many researchers who use the term "number sense" propose that we are born with the capacity to represent numerosities only approximately. It takes the acquisition of numerical symbols to represent numerosities exactly. I outline this position in Box 3.1.

Box 3.1 The analogue magnitude system

Following Dehaene and colleagues (Dehaene & Changeux, 1993), many researchers in this field have espoused the view that humans and other animals are not born with a number module that can represent sets and their numerosities. At best, they have an ability to represent numerosities only approximately.

The number of objects and the meaning of counting words (one, two, three …) are represented in the brain in an analogue way, hence this model is called the analogue magnitude system or the approximate number system. The internal (neural) representations of numbers is the same as the representation of continuous quantities, and that the internal (neural) representations of the numbers overlap and the more similar the numbers the more they overlap. This means that a set of four objects or the word four may sometimes be linked to the representation usually associated with fiveness or threeness, and less probably with the representations usually associated with sixness and twoness.

(*continued overleaf*)

The problems for this position have been well-rehearsed. It cannot support the basic properties of sets:

- the exact equivalence of two sets established by one-to-one correspondence because there are not sharp boundaries between the representation of the numbers
- the effects of adding or subtracting a member changes the numerosity of the set because this operation can only modify the probability that the representation will change the number

It has been argued that learning the counting words creates a qualitative change in the internal representations of numbers, both words and numerosities (Carey, 2009; Le Corre & Carey, 2007), though it is unclear how this happens.

A further problem arises from Dehaene's proposal and that is the logarithmic scaling of the internal representations. It is not possible mathematically to add or subtract numbers without transforming the log scaling into linear scaling.

Infant arithmetic

Possessing a concept of numerosity implies more than just being able to decide whether two sets do or do not have the same numerosity. It implies an ability to detect a change in numerosity when new members are added to the set, or old members away are taken away – in other words, to be able to compute the arithmetical consequences of adding and subtracting. Wynn (1992) showed that infants are able to do this, making use of the fact that babies look longer at events that violate their expectations. Infants of four to five months were shown a doll being placed on a stage, then covered by a screen, and then a second doll placed behind the screen. The infant could now see no dolls at all and had to imagine the situation behind the screen. If the infant had computed that one doll plus one doll makes two dolls, then her *arithmetical expectation* would be that there would be two dolls behind the screen. Wynn found that when the screen was removed, infants looked longer when there was one doll or three dolls than when there were two dolls. Similarly, when two dolls were placed on the stage, covered, and one doll shown to be removed, infants expected that there would be one doll left, and looked longer at other numbers.

This experiment has now been frequently replicated, and it has been shown that three to five month old infants look longer when the number of dolls is unexpected than when their identity is unexpected (i.e. one doll is surreptitiously changed behind the screen) (Simon et al., 1995). This shows that infants pay at least as much attention to the number of dolls as to their identity and visual properties.

Sequence of events 1+1 = 1 or 2

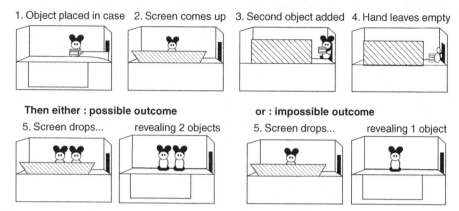

Figure 3.3 Infant addition. The infant sees the sequence of events in the top row, and then either a "possible outcome" where one doll added to one doll makes the two dolls shown; or an "impossible outcome" where the one doll added to one doll does not make two dolls. Bear in mind that the arithmetical operation has to take place in the head of the infant not in the displays. That is, the infant generates an arithmetical expectation of the outcome and if the display violates the expectation (the impossible outcome), the infant will look significantly longer at the display. Looking time is an indication of the arithmetical expectation.

Adapted from Wynn, 1992.

Sequence of events 2-1 = 1 or 2

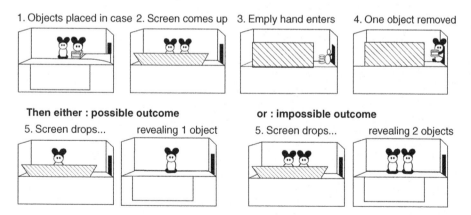

Figure 3.4 Infant subtraction. The infant sees one object being taken away, and then sees either the possible or impossible outcome. The infant generates an arithmetical expectation of the result of the subtraction. If the expectation is violated – the impossible outcome – this is signalled by the infant looking longer at the display.

Adapted from Wynn, 1992.

Learning the counting words

Counting aloud has the potential to make a bridge between the child's innate capacity for numerosity – the accumulator – to the more advanced mathematical achievements of the culture into which she was born. Though it seems very easy to us adults, learning to count takes about four years from two to six. Children start around two years old, and progress in stages until about six years old when they understand how to count and how to use counting in a near-adult manner.

The cultural context

Infants in a numerate society like ours begin to experience the culture of numbers very early on. Even before children could understand language, they would be exposed to games like counting fingers and toes; walking games like "One, two, three, hup!". Parents and carers will often count out objects, and ask children to do the same. They may talk about numbers and prices when they go shopping with their child. And then there are the stories we tell our children about three little piggies, seven dwarves, and so on. Or we recite nursery rhymes, that typically seem to involve numbers:

> *Sing a song of sixpence a pocket full of rye,*
> *Four and twenty blackbirds baked in a pie etc.*

> *One two buckle my shoe*
> *Three, four, knock at the door*
> *Five, six, pick up sticks*
> *Seven, eight, lay them straight*
> *Nine, ten, a big fat hen*
> *Eleven, twelve, dig and delve*
> *Thirteen, fourteen, maids a-courting*
> *Fifteen, sixteen, maids in the kitchen*
> *Seventeen, eighteen, maids in waiting*
> *Nineteen, twenty, my plate's empty*

> *One, two, three, four, five.*
> *Once I caught a fish alive,*
> *Six, seven, eight, nine, ten,*
> *Then I let it go again.*
> *Why did you let it go?*
> *Because it bit my finger so.*
> *Which finger did it bite?*
> *This little finger on the right.*

In fact, the more children experience numbers in the home, the better they will begin to learn arithmetic in school (Benavides-Varela et al., 2016).

One problem the child will face is that number words have several distinct meanings: numerosity, ordering, and labelling. "Three" can indicate the number of objects in a set, but it can also be used for ordering: *one, two, three, 1, 2, 3* for pages of a book, houses, places in a competition. Sometimes, special words are used for order: *first, second, third*. However, it easy to see that children learning about number can be confused about order and numerosity. Here's an example, from a three-year-old (Wynn, 1990)

> Experimenter (E): So how many are there? [A numerosity question]
> Adam (A): (counting three objects) One, two, five!
> E: (pointing towards the three items) So there's five here?
> A: No, *that's* five (pointing to the item he'd tagged "five"). One, two, five (counting them in the original order). [An order answer]

Of course, numerosity and order are closely related. Page 43 implies a set of 43 pages up to and including it, and we can order the numerosities by size: four comes after three and before five.

Labelling

We also use the same terms, mostly numerals, in a way that does not imply either numerosity or order. For example, a phone number, 4526289, isn't larger than 4526288 nor is there some kind of ordering of phone numbers from smaller to larger. TV Channel 2 and TV Channel 4 do not make TV Channel 6. Then there are bus routes, passport numbers (in the UK these are just nine numerals), and the ubiquitous barcodes.

Thus, the child learning to count and do arithmetic has to be able sort out the different meanings of number words. This seems to be a precondition for learning to use number words to help with the enumeration of sets, i.e. counting.

Principles of counting

The philosopher, John Locke, recognised that counting words are helpful in keeping in mind distinct large numerosities.

> Some Americans I have spoken with (who were otherwise of quick and rational parts enough) could not, as we do, by any means count to 1,000; nor had any distinct *idea* of that number, though they could reckon very well to 20.

These Americans, the "Tuoupinambos" (Tupinamba, in modern terminology) from the Brazilian jungle "lacked names for numbers above 5". Locke believed that we construct the idea of each number from the idea of "one" ("the most universal idea we have"). By repeating "this idea in our minds and adding the repetitions together … thus by adding [the idea of] of one to the [the idea of] one, we have the complex idea of a couple." He thought that number names were essential for acquiring distinct ideas of largish numbers, and that a *system* of number names "conduce[s] to well reckoning" (Locke, 1690/1961). Thus, for Locke, the basic ideas of numerosity are available to us without the help of culture, but that culture can be helpful in some circumstances.

Of course, Locke depended for this conclusion on casual observation rather than systematic investigation and modern methods have been used to explore this hypothesis in children raised in cultures that lacked names for numbers above five. Few such cultures still exist, in Amazonia, New Guinea and notably in Australia where few of the Aboriginal languages have number words above three, and those come through borrowing (Dixon, 1980). These studies broadly support Locke's contention that a system of number names is helpful for "well reckoning" (Butterworth et al., 2008; Pica et al., 2004)

Gelman and Gallistel in their classic book, *The Child's Understanding of Number*, have identified the competences, what they call "principles", that are required to be able to count, which are in some form innate (Gelman & Gallistel, 1978). This is sometimes called the *Principles Before* account of learning to count, which contrast with a view that children deduce or induce the principles from the practice of counting, the *Principles After* account (Butterworth & Reeve, 2012). *Principles Before* means that the child comes into the world equipped with something like the accumulator, since the principles are essentially implications or elaborations of the logic of the accumulator.

To illustrate the principles, consider the example of a child counting five dinosaurs:

- *The one-to-one principle*: each of these words must be linked with one and only one object: no word must be used more than once and all objects must be counted. That is, we must put each object in one–to–one correspondence with the counting words. This follows from one "cup" per object.
- *The cardinal principle*: the child must be in a position to announce the number of toy dinosaurs by using the last counting word used: "One, two, three, four, five. Five toy dinosaurs." This follows from the final level of the calibrated accumulator.
- *Abstractness*: which means that anything can be counted. The accumulator is neutral as to the nature of things counted.
- *Order-irrelevance*: which means that you can start counting with any object in the set and come up with same cardinality: one cup per object means that it is irrelevant which object you start with.

  In addition to these principles, there is the particular issue of the counting words themselves. For this is needed:
- *The stable order principle*: the child needs to know five counting words that are always in the same order – though they may not be *one, two three, four, five*. See "Adam" below.

As I suggested, a grasp of the principles follows from understanding the concept of numerosity. Sets are not intrinsically ordered. Understanding this means that you understand the order-irrelevance principle. There is also no constraint on the kinds of things that can be members of a set, provided they can be individuated. Understanding this implies holding the principle of abstractness. Of course, children and adults may possess the concept of numerosity and the accumulator mechanism with being able to fully implement the principles.

Learning the sequence of counting words

This is the first of these skills mastered. Children seem to know at about two and half what a number word is, and rarely intrude non-number words into the sequence, even when the order is incorrect (Fuson, 1988, Chapter 10).

Even learning the sequence of number words is not that straightforward. Children of two or three years often think of the first few number words as just one big word "onetwothreefourfive" and it takes them some time to learn that this big word is really five small words (Fuson, 1992).

Here is Adam, a three-and-a-half-year-old child, trying to count eight objects:

> One, two, three, four, eight, ten, eleben. No, try dat again. One, two, three, four, five, ten, eleben. No, try dat again. One! two! three-ee-four, five, ten, eleben. No. ... [finally] ... One, two, three, four, five, six, seven, eleven! Whew!
>
> (Gelman & Gallistel 1978)

This shows that even when the words are identified and separated getting the sequence right is a difficult stage.

One-to-one correspondence

This appears at about two years of age quite independently of learning the sequence of counting words. At two, children are able to give one sweet to each person, put one cup with each saucer and can name each person in a room or a picture, or point to them, once and only once (Potter & Levy, 1968). If you show a "puppet who is not very good at counting" counting the same object twice or missing an object altogether, children at three and a half are very good at spotting these violations of one-to-one correspondence (Gelman & Meck, 1983). And almost all children point to each object when they count, even when they can use the number words correctly, so there is one-to-one correspondence between objects, points and words (Gelman & Gallistel, 1978).

Children of three years or so may count in some but not all appropriate circumstances. When asked to give three toy dinosaurs, they may just grab a handful and give them to you without counting. Wynn calls them "Grabbers". Grabbers clearly know that number words represent a set of more than one, even if they have not yet grasped the role of number words in counting, and do not use the last word of a count to say how many (Wynn, 1990).

As we saw above in Wynn's Adam (not to be confused with Gelman and Gallistel's Adam), a child may think that the number word is just a *label* that attaches to an object.

In a give-a-number task, "Counters", children a few months older, will count, either aloud or silently, passing you the toys one by one. They also reliably give you the last word of the count in answer to "How many?" satisfying the cardinal principle. These children are initially able to count only small numerosities, and probably build up their competence systematically from one to two, from two to three, from three to four and so on up. In a give-a-number task, they will start by being able reliably to give one, then to give two, but perhaps not three, then three but perhaps not four. So by three and a half most children have a grasp of small numerosities, and know that counting is a way to find the numerosity of a set.

According to Gelman and her colleagues, children learning to count know the principles before their skills are fully developed. Certainly, children's performance is affected by number size, with larger numbers being harder (e.g. Fuson, 1988), and mastery of the three principles is not completely synchronised, with stable-order being reliably earliest, one-one correspondence between counting words and objects following later, and the cardinal principle the last of the three (Fuson, 1988, Chapter 10).

The cardinal word principle – the last number named in a count is the numerosity of the set counted – also follows from the concept of numerosity, since you are establishing a correlation between members of a set whose numerosity you do know, the number words up to five, say, and members of the set of things to be counted, whose numerosity you do not know. It may follow in a practical way as well. Recall that infants can recognise the numerosities of objects up to about three. Fuson suggests that children may notice that when they count a set "one two three", they get the same number as when they "subitize" the set (Fuson, 1988), which means being able to recognize the numerosity of the set without counting (see Chapter 4 for tests of subitizing and counting). This helps them realise that counting up to N is a way of establishing that a set has N objects in it. Repeating the count, and getting the same as the number obtained from subitizing, will reinforce the idea that every number name represents a unique numerosity. Again, this is something obvious to us, but may not be obvious to the child, especially as in practice the child will sometimes count the same set and get different results. He will count (or miscount) "one two three dinosaurs", and may count again, "one two four dinosaurs", and then again, "one two three four dinosaurs". He may wonder whether different number words can name the same numerosity, the numerosity of the set of dinosaurs.

Piaget (1952) was among the first to see that a full grasp of the concept of numerosity meant being able to abstract away from – ignore – irrelevant perceptual features of the set to be enumerated, so that you do not think, for example, there are more things just because they are more spread out (or more closely packed together). He saw the development of the child's thinking in general as a move away from the particular to the general and abstract.

Summary

- The human "starter kit" for learning school arithmetic includes two types of cognitive tool: domain-general, which can be applied to learning any school subject, and domain-specific – the "number module" - which is about sets and their numerosities and only applies to learning arithmetic.
- It is implemented, in part, by a simple accumulator mechanism.
- The child typically comes equipped with these tools, which provide the foundations for learning to count with words, and subsequently with symbols.
- The ability to use number words appropriately takes several years to accomplish

References

Anobile, G., Cicchini, G. M., & Burr, D. C. (2016). Number as a Primary Perceptual Attribute: A Review. *Perception*, 45, 5–31. doi: 10.1177/0301006615602599

Benavides-Varela, S., Butterworth, B., Burgio, F., Arcara, G., Lucangeli, D., & Semenza, C. (2016). Numerical Activities and Information Learned at Home Link to the Exact Numeracy Skills in 5–6 Years-Old Children. *Frontiers in Psychology*, 7(94). doi: 10.3389/fpsyg.2016.00094

Burr, D. C., & Ross, J. (2008). A visual sense of number. *Current Biology*, 18, 425–428.

Butterworth, B., & Reeve, R. (2012). Counting words and a principles-after account of the development of number concepts. In M. Siegal & L. Surian (Eds), *Access to Language and Cognitive Development*. Oxford: Oxford University Press.

Butterworth, B., Reeve, R., Reynolds, F., & Lloyd, D. (2008). Numerical thought with and without words: Evidence from indigenous Australian children. *Proceedings of the National Academy of Sciences of the USA*, 105, 13179–13184. doi: 10.1073_pnas.0806045105

Carey, S. (2009). Where our number concepts come from. *Journal of Philosophy*, 106(4), 220–254.

Cordes, S., Gelman, R., Gallistel, C. R., & Whalen, J. (2001). Variability signatures distinguish verbal from nonverbal counting for both large and small numbers. *Psychonomic Bulletin & Review*, 8(4), 698–707.

Dehaene, S., & Changeux, J.-P. (1993). Development of elementary numerical abilities: A neuronal model. *Journal of Cognitive Neuroscience*, 5, 390–407.

Dixon, R. M. W. (1980). *The Languages of Australia*. Cambridge: Cambridge University Press.

Fuson, K. C. (1988). *Children's Counting and Concepts of Number*. New York: Springer Verlag.

Fuson, K. C. (1992). Relationships between counting and cardinality from age 2 to 8. In J. Bideaud, C. Meljac, & J. P. Fisher (Eds), *Pathways to Number, Children's Developing Numerical Abilities*. Hillsdale, NJ: LEA.

Gelman, R., & Gallistel, C. R. (1978). *The Child's Understanding of Number* (1986 ed.). Cambridge, MA: Harvard University Press.

Gelman, R., & Meck, E. (1983). Preschoolers counting: Principles before skill. *Cognition*, 13, 343–359.

Hauser, M. D., Chomsky, N., & Fitch, W. T. (2002). The faculty of language: what is it, who has it, and how did it evolve? *Science*, 298, 1569–1579.

Izard, V., Sann, C., Spelke, E. S., & Streri, A. (2009). Newborn infants perceive abstract numbers. *Proceedings of the National Academy of Sciences*, 106(25), 10382–10385.

Jordan, K. E., & Brannon, E. M. (2006). The multisensory representation of number in infancy. *Proceedings of the National Academy of Sciences of the United States of America*, 103(9), 3486–3489.

Le Corre, M., & Carey, S. (2007). One, two, three, four, nothing more: An investigation of the conceptual sources of the verbal counting principles. *Cognition*, 105(2), 395–438. doi: 10.1016/j.cognition.2006.10.005

Leslie, A. M., Gelman, R., & Gallistel, C. R. (2008). The generative basis of natural number concepts. *Trends in Cognitive Sciences*, 12(6), 213–218. doi: 10.1016/j.tics.2008.03.004

Locke, J. (1690/1961). *An Essay concerning Human Understanding* (Based on Fifth Edition, edited by J. W. Yolton ed.). London: J. M. Dent.

Meck, W. H., & Church, R. M. (1983). A mode control model of counting and timing processes. *Journal of Experimental Psychology: Animal Behavior Processes*, 9(4), 320–334.

Pica, P., Lemer, C., Izard, V., & Dehaene, S. (2004). Exact and approximate calculation in an Amazonian indigene group with a reduced number lexicon. *Science*, 306, 499–503.

Pinker, S. (1994). *The Language Instinct*. London: Allen Lane The Penguin Press.

Pinker, S. (2008). *The Stuff of Thought. Language as a Window into Human Nature*. London: Penguin Books.

Potter, M. C., & Levy, E. I. (1968). Spatial enumeration without counting. *Child Development*, 39, 265–272.

Simon, T. J., Hespos, S. J., & Rochat, P. (1995). Do infants understand simple arithmetic? A replication of Wynn (1992). *Cognitive Development*, 10, 253–269.

Skorupski, P., MaBouDi, H., Galpayage Dona, H. S., & Chittka, L. (2018). Counting insects. *Philosophical Transactions of the Royal Society B: Biological Sciences*, 373(1740).

Wynn, K. (1990). Children's understanding of counting. *Cognition*, 36, 155–193.

Wynn, K. (1992). Addition and subtraction by human infants. *Nature*, 358, 749–751.

4

Core deficit in the number module

The cognitive cause of dyscalculia

LEVEL OF EXPLANATION	MEASURES	EDUCATIONAL CONTEXT
BEHAVIOURAL	Number sense Chapter 2	Society, school and home Chapter 8
COGNITIVE	Starter kit for learning arithmetic Chapter 3 **Core deficit as the cause of dyscalculia Chapter 4**	Assessment Chapter 9
	Development of arithmetic Chapter 5	Intervention Chapter 10
NEURAL	Brain structures and functions Chapter 6	Policy Chapter 11
GENETIC AND OTHER CAUSES Chapter 7		

I will argue that we inherit a *number module* that includes a *core capacity* for number abstraction and number reasoning. In Chapter 3, I showed how number sense underlies the development of arithmetical abilities, and outlined how other cognitive modules with their own core capacities – for example, language and colour perception – support extracting domain-specific information from the environment: that is, the modules are "tuned" to specific features of the environment and extract these features automatically. Now I turn to what happens when the number module fails to work efficiently which results in a *core deficit* in the capacity for number abstraction and number reasoning.

Core deficit

Let us consider a very large-scale study carried out by a department of the Organisation of Economic Cooperation and Development, and known as the PISA studies (not after the Italian city, but an acronym for the Programme for International

Student Assessment, which take place every three years). In 2012, around 510,000 students between the ages of 15 years 3 months and 16 years 2 months completed the assessment, representing about 28 million 15-year-olds in the schools of the 65 participating countries and economies.

Let us now consider what the norm could be. To be dyscalculic what percentile should the student be in on a standardized test of arithmetic: the lowest 10%, the lowest 5%, the lowest 25%? I could cite studies for each of these criteria, along with slightly fancier criteria in terms of standard deviation units.

In this study, 23% of students in OECD countries, and 32% of students in all participating countries and economies, *did not reach the baseline Level 2* in the PISA mathematics assessment. At that level, students can extract relevant information from a single source and can use basic algorithms, formulae, procedures or conventions to solve problems involving whole numbers. This is meant to be the minimum level a 15-year-old should be able to do in order to be a competent citizen.

The proportion of students below level 2 varies enormously from country to country (see Table 4.1).

Table 4.1 Proportion of 15–16-year-old children who failed to reach baseline Level 2 in mathematics.

Country	Average (%)
Singapore	8.3
Finland	12.3
UK	21.8
New Zealand	22.6
USA	25.8
Croatia	29.9
Morocco	75.7

Here's a level 2 question. Remember it is designed to test 15–16-year-olds:

Test Questions (Level 2) Helen The Cyclist

Helen has just got a new bike. It has a speedometer which sits on the handlebar.
    The speedometer can tell Helen the distance she travels and her average speed for a trip.

Question

On one trip, Helen rode 4 km in the first 10 minutes and then 2 km in the next 5 minutes.

Which one of the following statements is correct?

A. Helen's average speed was greater in the first 10 minutes than in the next 5 minutes.

B. Helen's average speed was the same in the first 10 minutes and in the next 5 minutes.

C. Helen's average speed was less in the first 10 minutes than in the next 5 minutes.

D. It is not possible to tell anything about Helen's average speed from the information given.

This means that what counts as the lowest *n*% will vary from country to country, and so the criterion or definition will depend on where the child is educated, *not their intrinsic numerical competence.*

What does it mean to have a core deficit?

Let's take an example from language to begin with. Now a small proportion of people are unable to learn language in the normal way because of a mutation in a gene (FOXP2) (Fisher et al., 1998). This mutation was inherited by members of the KE family who had deficits in several aspects of language processing. These included the production and comprehension of word inflections and syntactical structure, despite non-verbal abilities in the normal range. That is, they have a core deficit in the language module.

What about the "colour module"? There are some people who have *colour vision deficiency* ("colour blind" in popular discourse), by which is meant that they do not automatically see the world in colour in the way that most other people do. In most cases, the condition is inherited. For example, red-green colour-blindness is known to be due to a mutation on the X chromosome. Bear in mind that even the colour blind can often make the appropriate colour choices by using a *compensatory strategy.* For example, they can tell whether the traffic light is red or green by its position – red being top and green bottom, for example. That is, when the colour vision module is not working properly, they can resort to domain-general tools to try to do the same job. In the case of traffic lights, we could use our memory of what others have told us in language about location of the red, amber and green lights. Now this method may not be as efficient as seeing the colour of the lights, but it gets the job done.

My claim is that in some people, the number module is defective, just as it is in colour blindness or in specific language impairment. Perhaps a closer analogy is with *dyslexia.* A key mechanism in the language module is the ability to analyse speech sounds into their component and linguistically relevant parts, called "phonemes". That is, the language user can hear that the word "cat" contains three separate phonemes, the two consonants and the vowel. Now every speaker will say the word "cat" differently. Typically, children and women will pronounce the word with a higher pitch than an adult male; the volume of each occasion can be radically different, and exact acoustic properties of each sound will differ according to the shape of the speaker's vocal tract and their local "accent". Nevertheless, the language module enables the hearer to equate two very different acoustic signals as being instances of the same word containing the same three phonemes. This is called "categorical perception" where quite different acoustic signals are assigned to the same category, such as the k-category, the a-category or the t-category. (These linguistically relevant categories are conventionally written /k/, /t/, with *a* written /æ/ to distinguish it from other pronunciations of the letter *a* as in *alien*, *part*, and so on.)

Now, being able to do this is a requirement for learning to read in a language that uses an alphabetic script where each letter corresponds to a particular phoneme, and each phoneme is represented by a particular letter. Of course, most writing systems are full of exceptions to this one-to-one correspondence of letter to phoneme, English being the most notorious. However, being able to do this underpins how we typically learn to read these scripts. Now, if our language module is defective in doing this, then learning to read and write English will be very difficult, and will lead to the most common form of dyslexia (Snowling, 2000). This is a *core deficit* in the language module. Incidentally, if a language is not written alphabetically – such as Chinese or Japanese – then this core deficit will not prevent the dyslexic learning to read and write as well as anyone else. In fact, we carried out extensive tests on one boy whose parents were English-speakers but who was brought up in Japan. He was fully bilingual, and an excellent reader of Japanese (better than most of his Japanese classmates), but he was severely dyslexic in English (Wydell & Butterworth, 1999). (I deal with the relatively common co-occurrence of dyslexia and dyscalculia in Chapter 10.)

Now, there is an important difference between dyslexia and dyscalculia. There are no animal models of dyslexia because reading depends on language, and other species do not have anything like human language. It is possible to test whether animals have categorical perception of speech-like sounds, and indeed some species possess this for some speech sounds, such as the distinction between /t/ and /d/. This has been demonstrated in chinchillas (Kuhl, 1976), for example, but they are not able to integrate this capacity into learning words such as *time* and *dime*.

However, we know that many other species possess a number module (Agrillo & Beran, 2013). They can discriminate the numerosities of sets; they can identify a numerosity, say, four, and select a matching numerosity pattern, and in fact, monkeys use a similar brain network to humans (Nieder & Dehaene, 2009). This suggests that we humans share a specialized mechanism with our ancestors. I will deal with the question of heritability in more detail in Chapter 7.

Numbers and sets

The crucial arithmetical aspect of the number module is that numbers are inter-preted in terms of *sets*, upon which almost everything in number work is built. What this means in practice is that you find the very basis of number blindingly obvious – so obvious, in fact, that you don't even realise that you know it. By contrast dyscalculics may struggle with even the most basic numerical operations because they have failed to link operations on sets with the familiar arithmeti-cal operations. This can have the knock-on effect on the link between symbolic numbers – number words and digits – is not secure.

Here are some things that you know that dyscalculics may not know:

- Numbers are composed of other numbers: 4 can be composed of 1,1,1 and 1, or 2 and 2, etc. The parts of 4 are called "partitions" and there are 5 parti-tions of 4. These are very easy to see in terms of sets. □□□□□ can be bro-ken down into ones (□, □, □, □) into two subsets of two (□□,□□), etc.
- Addition is commutative: 3 + 5 is the same as 5 + 3

  □□□□ + □□□□□□   □□□□□□ + □□□□
- Addition and subtraction are inverse operations: if 5 + 3 = 8, then 8 − 5 = 3 and 8 − 3 = 5

  (□□□□□)□(□□□)
- Adding *n* to one addend in a sum means adding *n* to the total: 5 + 3 (+*n*) = 8 + *n*, e.g. 5 + 3 (+1) = 8 + 1
- The commutativity of multiplication follows from the interpretation as set 5 × 3 is the same 3 × 5:

  □□□□□   is the same as   □□□
  □□□□□   □□□
  □□□□□   □□□
                               □□□
                               □□□

What it's like to have a core deficit in the number module

What are the consequences of a deficit in the number module? Will it inevitably lead to a disability in learning arithmetic? Put it another way, is a deficit *sufficient* to cause a disability in learning arithmetic? We also need to consider the contrary case: are all difficulties and disabilities in learning arithmetic due to a deficit in the number module? That is, is it *necessary* to have a core deficit to have a disability in learning arithmetic? Bear in mind that I am talking just about numbers and arithmetic, not about other branches of mathematics. One of the dyscalculics we tested, Paul Moorcraft, managed to pass his maths exam because he was good at geometry – a big part of his curriculum – but was one of the most extreme cases of dyscalculia to come to our lab.

Dyscalculia is revealed in even the simplest numerical tasks. Remember Samantha Abeel, cited in Chapter 1: she said she couldn't tell the time, remember phone numbers, count money, balance her accounts, calculate the tip in restaurants, understand distances, and, more generally, "apply basic math to everyday life". When she was tested in the second grade, she was unable to subtract two from five, whether the numbers were presented as digits, $5 - 2 =$ ___, or concrete objects.

> Once again, my mom lays five cards in front of her.
> "OK, how many cards do I have in front of me?"
> I count them. "Five".
> "Good. Now how many do I have left after I take two away?"
> "But now you have three cards," I say again, bewildered and confused. I honestly do not understand.
>
> (Abeel, 2007, p. 17)

Even in the seventh grade, her problems persisted despite being a candidate for the Talented and Gifted class. She was unable to add two two-digit numbers in her head, to subtract from hundreds, to work out the value of a set of coins or identify the coins that would add up to $5.

This is entirely typical of dyscalculics. They can be normally competent, or even gifted in other domains, but still struggle with very simple numerical tasks. Like Abeel, they can be talented, hard-working, with support from parents and specialist teachers, and still not be able to do tasks that most of us take for granted.

This disability can have serious consequences. One of the first dyscalculics we tested was in prison for shoplifting. This was his solution for his inability to deal with numbers, and the sheer embarrassment and frustration involved in shopping. Would he have enough money to pay for the goods he wanted? How much should he offer at the till? Was he getting the right change? What would his friends or classmates think if they saw him so confused by this routine transaction?

In Abeel's case, she had trouble sleeping; and she avoided eating away from home because she would throw up so often. This had a dreadful effect on a young teenager's social life, as you may imagine. She was diagnosed with "panic attacks". These quickly disappeared when the school finally agreed to put her in a special education maths class instead of the regular seventh grade algebra class.

Annabel Cole learned to read early, did well at school and went on to read English at Cambridge University and now works as a national newspaper journalist. She described what it's like being dyscalculic:

> While words and language are the great love of my life, I've always been hopeless at maths. Ask me to tot up a shopping bill, or work out how to split the cost of a restaurant meal, and I break out in a cold sweat. In the classroom, my one academic blackspot was maths: my inability to grasp even the most basic principles filled me with horror and shame.

Memories of my primary school in Edinburgh are haunted by one particular teacher who would scream at me, in front of the class, on a daily basis. At secondary school I was in the bottom set for maths, but somehow scraped a C in my GCSE, with an awful lot of help and cramming.

However, my ineptitude has been far more burdensome in adult life. To this day, I can't write out numbers longer than four digits (tell me that something costs £25,000 and I'll struggle to express that as a figure) and have no idea how to grasp the breakdowns on utility bills or work out supermarket special offers.

I must be the only person in Britain who was relieved when my cleaner's rate of pay went up from £8 to £10 an hour, making her wages easier to calculate. I even put the wrong number of candles on a birthday cake for one of my daughters when she turned five.

My problem is not confined to calculations. I find timings hard and get dates wrong. Yet it never crossed my mind there might be something wrong with me. Family and friends said: "You can't be good at everything." That's what I thought, too.

(*Daily Mail*, 27.11.2015)

Dyscalculia on Facebook is full of similar stories. Debbie Moore writes,

I grew up with undiagnosed Dyscalculia…. My school years were a hellish nightmare because of it. I had no self esteem, struggled socially, and failed Arithmetic and Math from 1st grade onward. I excelled in Reading and English, which only made things worse. I was constantly humiliated and belittled by my parents, teachers and classmates. I was told I did so bad in Math because I chose to hate the subject. I wanted to become a Veterinarian or a Pediatrician which of course was impossible because I couldn't understand any Math. I would get laughed at by everyone, including my teachers and parents, and was told I'd amount to nothing. I was forced to attend summer school every damn summer, which I hated with a passion. I used to feel sick to my stomach every morning before school. I had countless sleepless nights worrying about the next day of school…. Nothing made me happier while I was filling in all the questionnaires for [my son], when I recognized that I had all the signs of Dyscalculia that he was diagnosed with! If I had won the lottery that day I couldn't have been happier!

I will return to the problem of labelling in Chapter 10 on assessment, but I have countless stories of adults and children who are just relieved to know that they have this specific learning disability and are not just stupid. Being labelled as dyscalculic is much better than being labelled as stupid. I recently received an email from a 45-year-old woman who has had a lifetime of distress with numbers: "Even just a name for what I have" would help.

In fact, many children disguise their disability – which they attribute to their own stupidity – by misbehaving. Here's what one teacher told us:

> lots of times they're trying to cover it up. And sometimes they'll cover it up – they'd rather be told off for being naughty than being told off that they're thick.

Our own research documents very similar stories in both adults and children.

Ben, a very bright eight-year-old, who was good at, and enjoyed all, school subjects, including science, and had expert knowledge of dinosaurs, was unable to do very simple tasks such as finding how much you need to add to 8 to make 30, even with the aid of units and tens number blocks (from *Sorry, Wrong Number* ... a film by Butterworth & Gabbay).

We used focus groups to find out what nine-year-old dyscalculics thought of their daily numeracy hour. Focus groups seemed to Anna Bevan, my wonderfully insightful student and research assistant on this project, the best way to go, because even at nine, children know what to say to adults. So, if you ask them whether they like maths, they'll invariably say Yes, and they will tell you that they like their teacher and that they are getting on well in the maths lessons. When you put low-attaining learners together, they start to talking to each other more than to the adult moderator, and this can be more revealing. We divided the children into three types of group – high, middle, and low-attaining – according to teacher ratings and our own tests. One question concerned how well they understood the topic the teacher introduced at the beginning of the lesson (Bevan & Butterworth, 2007). We recorded every group and then transcribed them verbatim. Here's what some of the children said.

> Child 2: I sometimes don't understand whatever she (the teacher) says.
> Child 2: I don't forget it, I don't even know what she's saying.
> Child 3: When you listen to the teacher, then you turn your head and you don't know nothing.... If I remember something, and then the teacher says "stop for a second, just listen to me" then as soon as she talks, yeah, and we come back, we do work, and I say "what do I have to do?" I always forget.
> Child 4: Somebody says "can you pass me – can you pass the rubber?" "Can you pass the pencil?" "Can you pass the pencil sharpener?" and what are you supposed to do? I'm trying to work out and you lose track. You have to do it over and over again and by the time you're finished you've just done the first question and the teacher says "why have you only done one question?"

We also asked about their emotional responses to the maths lessons, and I'll deal with that in Chapter 10 on intervention.

Memory for numerical information

Our low-attaining focus group participants frequently talked about forgetting. Here's an example

> Child 1: You might forget what the teacher has taught you.

Teachers of course also noticed that the dyscalculic children forget most, or all, of what they've been taught, and that this creates a real problem for the teacher:

> KD: If they forget really basic things from the beginning, then there's no way you can use those further down the line, so if they're really struggling with taking away, and knowing it's the difference or whatever, you can't do exchanging or whatever because it's – they can't even do the basics.

A defective number module means that remembering number facts is difficult, and most dyscalculics report that they have trouble not only with arithmetical facts but also with non-arithmetical number facts, such as their PINs, dates and times. Memorizing something new is easy if you already have a meaningful structure into which it will fit. For example, it is easy to remember quite a long sentence. In one of our studies, listeners could recall perfectly a sentence of 30 words on one hearing under appropriate conditions (Wingfield & Butterworth, 1984). Words in a sentence are easier to remember than a sequence of unrelated words because we have a mental mechanism designed to understand and retain meaningful sentences. By contrast, it is hard to recall accurately more than seven unrelated words, letters or digits. And recalling words of a foreign language – much less meaningful – is harder still, with a limit of about three items. Meaningfulness and structure is even more important for long-term memory (Baddeley, 1986; Butterworth et al., 1990).

If numbers have little meaning for dyscalculics, they are going to have trouble remembering them because they will not fit into a meaningful existing mental structure. They are just words. Now they may be able to repeat back a sequence such as "six nines are fifty-four" but they are unlikely to be able to remember this sequence the next day.

Testing for a core deficit

We saw in Chapter 2 average performance and also individual differences in three ways for assessing domain-specific capacities in number sense:

- Accuracy of magnitude comparison (comparing two dot arrays)
- Speed and accuracy of dot enumeration (saying the number of dots)
- Accuracy of marking a number line.

We also saw that these measures were good predictors of how well a learner would learn arithmetic. We also saw that all learners improved with age on these measures but the relative difference remained fairly stable, where it was measured in the same way in the same child over time.

Dot enumeration

The clearest example of this is in a longitudinal study using dot enumeration carried out in Melbourne, Australia, with my colleagues there, Robert Reeve, Fiona Reynolds and Judi Humberstone. We examined how quickly and how accurately the children could name the number of dots. We then explored four parameters of their performance (see Figure 4.1, which we first saw in Box 2.1).

In our longitudinal study each child was re-tested using the same test at four ages, and for each child their performance was compared with their age-matched peers on the four parameters. This meant we could ask:

■ Is child X better or worse than his or her peers?
■ Does child X remain better or worse than his or her peers.

For worse or better, we did not use arbitrary criteria – such as below or above a particular percentile – but cluster analysis to see if there really were different clusters, or groups, of learners. It turned out that testing five times between kindergarten and 11 years revealed three clusters at each age, which we termed Slow, Medium and Fast. Children tended to stay within the same cluster. I show the results in Figure 4.2.

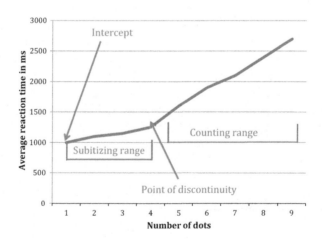

Figure 4.1 The parameters of dot enumeration: (1) the Reaction Time (RT) slope within the subitizing range; (2) the RT slope for the counting range; (3) the subitizing range (indicated by the point of slope discontinuity); and (4) the overall average RT. The intercept is the RT for One, and is an indicator of individual differences in basic RT. In adults, for items in the subitizing range (1 to 4) the slope function is typically shallow (increments of between 40–120 msecs per item; in the counting range the increment tends to be 250–350 msecs per item).

Trick & Pylyshyn, 1993.

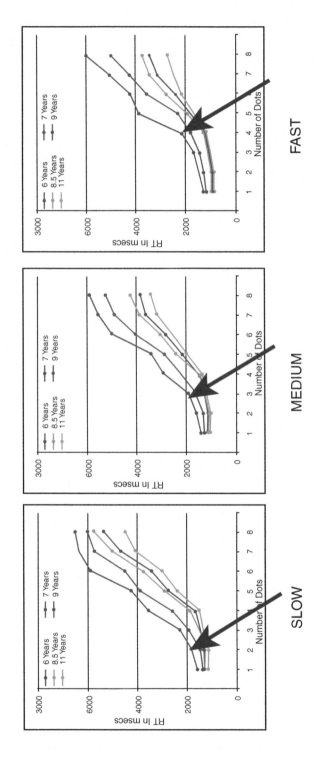

Figure 4.2 Dot enumeration of profiles of 159 learners from kindergarten (up to six years) to 11 years. The arrows indicate the subitizing range in kindergarten: the Slow cluster subitized two items, the Medium three, and the Fast four. By eight and a half years all were subitizing four items.

From Reeve, Reynolds, Humberstone, & Butterworth, 2012.

Children in the Slow cluster in kindergarten were only able to subitize two items, while the Medium were already able to subitize three and the Fast four; but by eight and a half years all were in the adult range subitizing four items. Cluster membership predicted accuracy in age appropriate arithmetic from kindergarten single-digit addition to two-digit addition, subtraction and multiplication at nine and a half years, and three digit subtraction, multiplication and division at ten years. Just to be clear, other cognitive factors did not define the three clusters. So, for example, the Slow group were not slow on other tasks. We also assessed all the children with a standard test of nonverbal reasoning (Raven's Coloured Progressive Matrices (Raven et al., 1995)); again there were no significant differences between the Slow and the other two clusters (Reeve et al., 2012). See Chapter 5 for more on domain-general cognitive factors.

This is the longest and most detailed longitudinal study of arithmetical development so far published.

We have also mined these data for other evidence that dot enumeration is linked to calculation fluency and to understanding the principles of arithmetic. I'll say more about this in the next chapter, Chapter 5, on the development of arithmetic.

Dot enumeration and the prevalence of dyscalculia

Dot enumeration has been used in a large prevalence study in Cuba led by Vivian Reigosa Crespo and Mitchell Valdes Sosa at the Cuban Centre for Neuroscience (Reigosa-Crespo et al., 2012). With this study we could first estimate the proportion of children who were dyscalculic, using this theoretically motivated measure. In this study, we started with every child from 6.9 to 17.3 in one district of Havana, 11562 of them, all of whom underwent a curriculum-based group-administered standardized test each school year – see MAT in Figure 4.3, where you can also see our sampling methods and results. Of these, 1966 were tested individually using a specially designed computerized "basic numerical battery" (BNB) comprising the following measures of efficiency that combined accuracy and speed (median RT adjusted for basic RT/accuracy). This is called "inverse efficiency" (IE) since the higher the score the lower the efficiency.

- Item-timed arithmetic (IE) – the measure of arithmetical competence.
- Item-timed dot enumeration (IE) – the measure of core numerical capacity
- Basic reaction time so we could establish whether the learner was slow on everything or just on the number tests.

Of the 1966 tested, 9.4% were classified as Arithmetic Dysfluent (AD), meaning that they were 2 s.d. worse on timed arithmetic; 4.5% were classified as having a Core Deficit based on their performance on dot enumeration; and 3.4% were classified as Developmental Dyscalculic (DD) if they were both AD and had a core deficit (see Figure 4.3).

This approach allows us to ask another question, and a very important one at that. Is a core deficit *sufficient* for arithmetical dysfluency (AD)? That is, if a learner

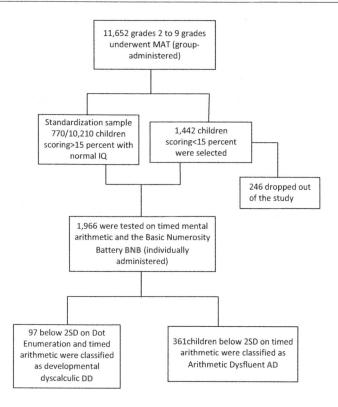

Figure 4.3 The structure of the Havana prevalence study.

Adapted from Reigosa-Crespo et al., 2012.

has a core deficit will they necessarily have difficulty learning arithmetic? The answer is a definite Yes. That is, having a core deficit makes it almost certain that a child will have difficulty in being normally fluent in arithmetic. Incidentally, the standardized school test, MAT, is actually a much less good predictor of which child is going to have trouble and which not. (Technically, in terms of the *specificity* of the core deficit test (true negative (1570)/true negative + false positive (35)), the true–negative rate is 98%, positive predictive value 74% and negative predictive value 86%. While in terms of the *sensitivity* of the core-deficit test, the true–positive rate is 27%; that is, there are many causes of AD besides the core deficit.)

Hearing about this Havana study, the then president of Cuba, Fidel Castro, asked for a national survey be undertaken, and for it to include tests for dyslexia and ADHD, as well as their test for dyscalculia. For the Cuban National Survey of Learning Disabilities, my Cuban colleagues trained 240 specialists (psychologists, speech therapists, psychiatrists, and teachers) to carry out the individual testing on a representative sample of over 16,000 children from Grades 3 to 6 from 270 schools across Cuba. This study confirmed the prevalence estimate of 3–4% for dyscalculia, and found prevalences of 4.3% for dyslexia and 9.4% for ADHD.

These Cuban studies are by far the largest studies of dyscalculia carried out anywhere.

Other estimates suggest a *prevalence* of dyscalculia using a number sense as well as a calculation criterion is somewhere between 3.5% and 7% of the population. This accords with an earlier survey by the Israeli paediatrician Ruth Shalev (Shalev, 2007) who used a different criterion – two years behind peers on a standardized test of arithmetic.

Charles

One of the first dyscalculics we tested formally with dot enumeration was Charles. He was in his late twenties, and a psychology graduate. This meant that he had managed to pass the statistics component of his degree. This component involved learning how to use a computer stats package by following a kind of recipe for tabulating data and selecting the appropriate test. Understanding underlying concepts is not required. In fact, I suspect many of my non-dyscalculic students don't understand the basis of the stats they are using. We tested Charles on dot enumeration and compared his results with matched controls. The results are presented in Figure 4.4.

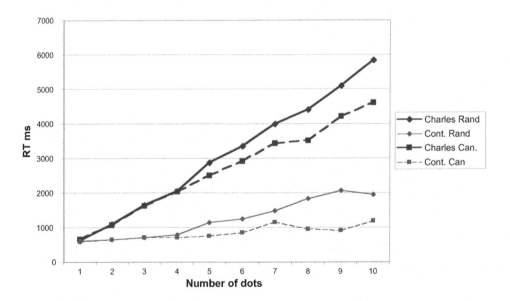

Figure 4.4 Charles's timed dot enumeration. We used both random dot arrays ("Rand" in the Figure) and also "canonical" dot arrays ("can" in the Figure) which are the familiar playing card patterns. "Cont." are the non-dyscalculic age and education matched controls. Unsurprisingly, non-dyscalculics adults and children are faster to name the number of dots in the canonical arrays (Mandler & Shebo, 1982). Charles was also faster for these arrays, but, overall, he was very much slower for all numerosities above 1 dot.

Koontz and Berch: matching dots and digits

This is another early study, and one of the first to look at poor number sense as a cause of "arithmetic learning disability" (ALD) which meant in the bottom 25% of the age group. Here ten-year-olds had to decide whether two or three dots matched the digits 2 or 3 as quickly as possible, a very easy task but one which produced more errors and was answered more slowly in the ALD group than in a matched control group (Koontz & Berch, 1996).

Now ALD isn't the same as dyscalculia, though a group defined as being in the bottom 25% is likely to contain some dyscalculics. The reason for this is that the bottom 25% will contain learners who do poorly on standard tests of arithmetic for a wide variety of causes. A child who misses a lot of lessons could well be ALD but not dyscalculic, for example. The Havana study suggests that the prevalence of dyscalculia is much less than 25%.

Geary's Number Sets test

Another prospective longitudinal study had similar findings to the study by Reeve et al. This study used a task called *Number Sets* as a way of measuring number sense (see Figure 4.5). In this task children in first-grade had to identify small sets of dots, or a combination of two sets of dots, that added up to a target number of 5 or less (Geary et al., 2009) (see Figure 4.5). About 6% of the children were identified by later tests as having "Mathematical Learning Disability". It turned out that performance on Number Sets predicted which of these children would be in this group. Like the study by Reeve et al, IQ was not a predictor. Again, we find that dysfunctional number sense is sufficient to cause a disability in learning arithmetic.

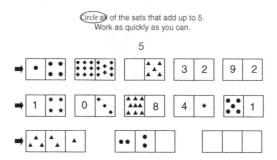

Figure 4.5 Number sets test. "There are four pages of such items, and the child is instructed to move across each line of the page from left to right without skipping any and to 'circle any groups that can be put together to make the top number, five ([or]nine)' and to 'work as fast as you can without making many mistakes.' The child is given 60s and 9s per page for the targets 5 and 9, respectively, and is asked to stop at the time limit" (Geary et al., 2009, p. 416).

It is important to ensure that your measures are really measuring something real, not a simple artefact of the measuring tool. We call this "construct validity". It is true that both dot enumeration and Number Sets give corroborating results, but they are very similar tests in that they involve both symbols – number words or digits – and a set of objects. In the case of dot enumeration, the learner produces a number word to designate the number of objects in a set, in Number Sets, some items require matching a digit to a set.

In these studies, the learner has to link the numerosity of the set, or sets, to a number word or a digit. It has been suggested that the dyscalculic disability is not caused by a deficit in number sense – the number abstraction capacity of the number module – but rather a difficulty in linking number sense to these cultural tools. One study by Belgian psychologist, Pascale Noël and colleagues found that seven- and eight-year-olds seemed to have typical number sense but were significantly worse than their peers in comparing numbers (Rousselle & Noël, 2007). In a later study, these authors found that ten- and 11-year-old dyscalculics did indeed have a deficit in number sense (Mussolin et al., 2010).

Magnitude comparison test

Another type of study does not involve the person in linking counting words or digits to the numerosity of sets, as I mentioned in Chapter 2. Here all that is required is to select the set with more objects. Even fish can do this. However, there are important individual differences in how well this is done. One study by Italian psychologist Manuela Piazza and colleagues linked individual differences in this task with dyscalculia. Dyscalculics were identified using a standard Italian clinical measure. (Piazza et al., 2010)

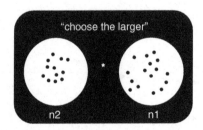

Figure 4.6 The task is to select the disk with most dots. The lower panel shows the ability to discriminate in terms of the proportional difference between the two: that is, the more similar the numbers the more difficult it is to make the discrimination accurately. As you can see, this ability improves with age. The ten-year-old dyscalculics performed at the same level as five-year-olds.

From Piazza et al., 2010.

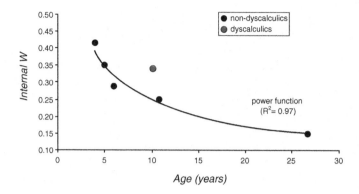

Figure 4.6 (*Continued*)

Summary

- A *core deficit* in the number module – the ability to abstract the numerosity of sets – is linked to profound and life-long difficulties with number.
- It is straightforward to identify this deficit using a task like timed dot enumeration.

References

Abeel, S. (2007). *My Thirteenth Winter: A Memoir*. NYC, NY: Scholastic.

Agrillo, C., & Beran, M. J. (2013). Number without language: comparative psychology and the evolution of numerical cognition. *Frontiers in Psychology*, 4.

Baddeley, A. D. (1986). *Working Memory*. Oxford: Clarendon Press.

Bevan, A., & Butterworth, B. (2007). *The responses to maths disabilities in the classroom*. Draft 2002. Retrieved from www.mathematicalbrain.com/pdf/2002BEVANBB.PDF

Butterworth, B., Shallice, T., & Watson, F. (1990). Short-term retention of sentences without "short-term memory". In G. Vallar & T. Shallice (Eds), *Neuropsychological Impairments of Short-Term Memory*. Cambridge: Cambridge University Press.

Fisher, S. E., Vargha-Khadem, F., Watkins, K. E., Monaco, A. P., & Pembrey, M. E. (1998). Localisation of a gene implicated in a severe speech and language disorder. *Nature Genetics*, 18(2), 168–170.

Geary, D. C., Bailey, D. H., Littlefield, A., Wood, P., Hoard, M. K., & Nugent, L. (2009). First-grade predictors of mathematical learning disability: A latent class trajectory analysis. *Cognitive Development*, 24, 411–429.

Koontz, K. L., & Berch, D. B. (1996). Identifying simple numerical stimuli: processing inefficiencies exhibited by arithmetic learning disabled children. *Mathematical Cognition*, 2(1), 1–23.

Kuhl, P. K. (1976). Speech perception by the chinchilla: Categorical perception of synthetic alveolar plosive consonants. *The Journal of the Acoustical Society of America*, 60(S1), S81–S81. doi: 10.1121/1.2003550

Mandler, G., & Shebo, B. J. (1982). Subitizing: An analysis of its component processes. *Journal of Experimental Psychology: General*, 11, 1–22.

Mussolin, C., Mejias, S., & Noël, M.-P. (2010). Symbolic and nonsymbolic number comparison in children with and without dyscalculia. *Cognition*, 115(1), 10–25. doi: 10.1016/j.cognition.2009.10.006

Nieder, A., & Dehaene, S. (2009). Representation of Number in the Brain. *Annual Review of Neuroscience*, 32(1), 185–208. doi: 10.1146/annurev.neuro.051508.135550

Piazza, M., Facoetti, A., Trussardi, A. N., Berteletti, I., Conte, S., Lucangeli, D., Dehaene, S., & Zorzi, M. (2010). Developmental trajectory of number acuity reveals a severe impairment in developmental dyscalculia. *Cognition*, 116(1), 33–41.

Raven, J. C., Court, J. H., & Raven, J. (1995). *Coloured Progressive Matrices*. Oxford, UK: Oxford Psychologists Press.

Reeve, R., Reynolds, F., Humberstone, J., & Butterworth, B. (2012). Stability and Change in Markers of Core Numerical Competencies. *Journal of Experimental Psychology: General*, 141(4), 649–666. doi: 10.1037/a0027520

Reigosa-Crespo, V., Valdes-Sosa, M., Butterworth, B., Estevez, N., Rodriguez, M., Santos, E., … Lage, A. (2012). Basic Numerical Capacities and Prevalence of Developmental Dyscalculia: The Havana Survey. *Developmental Psychology*, 48(1), 123–135. doi: 10.1037/a0025356

Rousselle, L., & Noël, M.-P. (2007). Basic numerical skills in children with mathematics learning disabilities: A comparison of symbolic vs non-symbolic number magnitude processing. *Cognition*, 102(3), 361–395.

Shalev, R. S. (2007). Prevalence of developmental dyscalculia. In D. B. Berch & M. M. M. Mazzocco (Eds), *Why is Math so Hard for Some Children? The Nature and Origins of Mathematical Learning Difficulties and Disabilities* (pp. 49–60). Baltimore, MD: Paul H Brookes Publishing Co.

Snowling, M. J. (2000). *Dyslexia*. Oxford: Blackwell.

Wingfield, A., & Butterworth, B. (1984). Running memory for sentences: syntactic parsing as a control function in working memory. In H. Bouma & D. Bouwhuis (Eds), *Attention and Performance* (Vol. X). Hillsdale, NJ: Erlbaum.

Wydell, T. N., & Butterworth, B. (1999). A case study of an English-Japanese bilingual with monolingual dyslexia. *Cognition*, 70, 273–305.

5

Development of arithmetic depends on domain-specific numerical competences

LEVEL OF EXPLANATION	MEASURES	EDUCATIONAL CONTEXT
BEHAVIOURAL	Number sense Chapter 2	Society, school and home Chapter 8
COGNITIVE	Starter kit for learning arithmetic Chapter 3 Core deficit as the cause of dyscalculia Chapter 4	Assessment Chapter 9
	Development of arithmetic Chapter 5	Intervention Chapter 10
NEURAL	Brain structures and functions Chapter 6	Policy Chapter 11
	GENETIC AND OTHER CAUSES Chapter 7	

In Chapter 2, I discussed the development of number sense, and showed how it is possible to measure it even in infants. Research demonstrated that individual differences in number sense are statistically related to the development of arithmetic and, as I showed in Chapter 3, the critical idea here is that arithmetic is based on a core capacity for understanding the *numerosity of a set* – that is, the number of objects in a set. This, I proposed, is a necessary tool in the *starter kit* for the development of arithmetic. In Chapter 4, I showed how a *core deficit* in this capacity is at the root of dyscalculia. In this chapter, I discuss in more detail with how the core capacity for representing numerosities underlies the development of arithmetic.

Back to basics

To understand how tools in the *starter kit* mould the development of arithmetic, we must first be clear about the nature of arithmetic itself. The psychologists, Rochel Gelman and Charles Gallistel make an important distinction in their classic study *The Child's Understanding of Number*. On the one hand, there is the child's *number-abstraction* abilities, which are used to abstract specific or relative numerosity (see below) from a display. For example, the child will be able to tell that a collection has a particular number of objects, for example, that there are five apples on the table, and also that there are as many apples and bananas, or that there are more in one collection than in the other. The child will have *number-reasoning abilities* that supports inferences about the transformations on the collection, for example, will rearrangement change the numerosity; and what will be the effect of other operations on the collections, such as combining them.

All readers will know what I am about to describe, but may not be aware that they know it, or have forgotten that they know it.

Arithmetic is based on sets

The type of collection that underpins arithmetic is the *set*. A set has a definite number of members, which I will call its *numerosity*. Numerosity is an abstract property of the set since two sets of quite different types of thing can have the same numerosity, such as the number of fingers on my left hand and the number of chimes of Big Ben at five o'clock. My fingers and the chimes have nothing in common apart from their number. You can also have a set of sets, such as the set of the sets of fingers on both of my hands, or the set of the set of my fingers and the set of chimes, which is a set with numerosity fifteen. The reason I stress the abstractness of numerosities is because this will be important in learning arithmetic.

Reasoning about numerosities follows from their basis in sets. The child must be able to infer that some operations on sets change the numerosity, such as adding a member or taking away a member, and other operations, such as rearranging the members, does not change the numerosity, but rather "conserves" it.

Further inferences, usually later in development, will be based on operation of taking the *union* of sets. For example, $3 + 5 = 8$ can be explained as the union of two sets (they have to be separate or "disjoint") with numerosities 3 and 5. The result of the union is a set that has the numerosity 8. Similarly, the other arithmetical operations – subtraction, multiplication and division – can be explained in terms of sets

The key point is that arithmetic is based sets and, as we will see below, most informal and formal educational approaches to learning the counting words uses sets of concrete objects, and teaching arithmetic usually starts with sets of concrete objects, and manipulations of them – making the union of sets for addition, taking away subsets to indicate subtraction.

Piaget's reasoning tools

According to the psychologist, Jean Piaget, the child goes through stages of cognitive development, which become increasingly sophisticated, general and abstract.

For Piaget, children progressively reorganize operations on their thoughts ("schemas") and cognitive processes in response to their experiences of the environment, by "assimilating" new experiences to existing schemas, or modifying the schema ("accommodation") when it fails to fit the new experience.

He proposed four distinct stages of cognitive development:

- sensori–motor (birth–two years) when the child understands the world only through perceptions and action
- pre-operational (two to seven years) can represent the world through mental images and language
- concrete operational (seven–12 years) when the child begins to reason logically and can represent the world in categories
- formal operations (12 years onwards), the child can generate hypotheses and test them

At each stage, reasoning tools the child has available are applied to the development of a wide range of concepts, including what he called "the concept of number" (Piaget, 1952). To possess this concept, the necessary preconditions were a grasp of certain logical principles, since numbers are really a part of logic:

> Our hypothesis is that the construction of number goes hand-in-hand with the development of logic, and that a pre-numerical period corresponds to a pre-logical level. Our results do, in fact, show that number is organized, stage after stage, in close connection with gradual elaboration of systems of inclusion (hierarchy of logical classes) and systems of asymmetrical relations (qualitative seriations), the sequence of numbers thus resulting from an operational synthesis of classification and seriation. In our view, logical and arithmetical operations therefore constitute a single system that is psychologically natural, the second resulting from a generalization and fusion of the first, under two complementary headings of inclusion of classes and seriation of relations, quality being disregarded.
>
> (Piaget, 1952. viii)

Thus, for Piaget, the "concept of number", (which corresponds to our idea of "numerosity"), is built on more basic and *more general* capacities available initially in the concrete operational stage. These included the capacity to reason transitively; that is, the child should be able to reason from the facts that if A is bigger than B, and B is bigger than C, then A is bigger than C. Without this capacity, the child could not put the numbers in order of size, which is clearly fundamental. A second capacity the child must develop, is the idea that the number of things in a set is "conserved", to use his technical term, unless a new object is added to the set, or an object subtracted from it. Merely moving the objects around – should not affect number: for example, spreading them out so they take up more room. Even more basic than either of these two capacities, as Piaget pointed out, is the ability to abstract away from the perceptual properties of the things in the set, and not be seduced by physical appearances. To grasp the numerosity of a set, one needs to ignore all the particular features of the objects in it – their colour, their shape, their size, and even what they are: a set of three cats has the same numerosity as a set of three chairs, or indeed of three wishes. The idea of number is abstract. And the ideas of the "same number" or "different numbers" are abstractions from abstractions. The emergence of the capacity for numerosity will depend on the development of the necessary prior capacities, what Piagetians call "prerequisites". It will also depend, as do many conceptual and logical abilities, on interacting with the world. The concept of numerosity could emerge as a result of manipulating objects, for example, lining up sets to establish one-to-one correspondence between the members of the two sets, for sharing out sweets or toys.

One problem with Piaget's approach is that the infant cannot have a concept of number since the reasoning tools only become available – as a result of maturation and interaction with environment – when the child reaches seven years old, or thereabouts. So it cannot be in the starter kit. In fact, infants can and do have arithmetical capacities.

To recap: possessing a concept of numerosity implies more than just being able to decide whether two sets do or do not have the same numerosity. It implies an ability to detect a change in numerosity when new members are added to the set, or old members away are taken away – in other words, to be able to compute the arithmetical consequences of adding and subtracting. Wynn (1992) showed that infants are able to do this, making use of the fact that babies look longer at events that violate their expectations. Infants of four to five months were shown a doll being placed on a stage, then covered by a screen, and then a second doll placed behind the screen (see Chapter 3). The infant could now see no dolls at all and had to imagine the situation behind the screen. If the infant had computed that one doll plus one doll makes two dolls, then her *arithmetical expectation* would be that there would be two dolls behind the screen. Wynn found that when the screen was removed, infants looked longer when there was one doll or three dolls than when there were two dolls. Similarly, when two dolls were placed on the stage, covered, and one doll shown to be removed, infants expected that there would be one doll left, and looked longer at other numbers (see Figure 3.4 in Chapter 3).

Understanding arithmetic

Counting is the basis of arithmetic for most children. Since the result of adding two numerosities is equivalent to counting the union of two disjoint sets with those numerosities, children can learn about adding by putting two sets together and counting the members of their union.

From counting all to counting on

Children make use of their counting skills in the early stages of learning arithmetic. The number words, as was noted in the Introduction, have both a sequence (ordinal) and a numerosity (or cardinal) meaning. As Fuson and Kwon point out, "In order for number words to be used for addition and subtraction, they must take on cardinal meanings" (Fuson & Kwon, 1992, p. 291). Children often represent the numerosity of the addend by using countable objects, especially fingers, to help them think about and solve arithmetical problems.

There appear to be three main stages in the development of counting as an addition strategy:

1. Counting all. For 3 + 5, children will count "one, two, three" and then "one, two, three, four, five" countables to establish the numerosity of the sets to be added, so that two sets will be made visible – for example, three fingers on one hand and five fingers on the other. The child will then count all the objects.
2. Counting on from first. Some children come to realise that it is not necessary to count the first addend. They can start with three, and then count on another five to get the solution. Using finger counting, the child will no longer count out the first set, but start with the word "Three", and then use a hand to count on the second addend: "Four, five, six, seven, eight".
3. Counting on from the larger number. It is more efficient, and less prone to error, when the smaller of the two addends is counted. The child now selects the larger number to start with: "Five", and then carries on "Six, seven, eight".

(Butterworth, 1999; Carpenter & Moser, 1982)

The stages are not strictly separate, in that children may shift strategies from one problem to the next. There is a marked shift to Stage 3 in the first six months of school (around five to six years old in the US, where this study was conducted (Carpenter & Moser, 1982)). Stage 3 shows a grasp of the fact that taking the addends in either order will give the same result. This may follow from an understanding of the effects of joining two sets, that is, taking the union of two disjoint sets.

Even in the earliest phases of the development of addition abilities, children do not need to count the union of the sets. In one set of experiments, Starkey and Gelman showed the children two sets one at a time so that there was no opportunity to count all the elements. In these circumstances, most three-year-olds could solve 2+1, and a few could solve 4 + 2. By five years, all could solve the first and 81% the second. Interestingly, only 56% solved 2 + 4, suggesting that some of the children were not counting on from larger, but were still counting on from first (Starkey & Gelman, 1982).

From counting on to arithmetical facts

The skilled adult typically will not need to calculate or count single digit problems such as $3 + 5$, 3×5, $5 - 3$, or $6 \div 3$ and will simply retrieve the solution from memory.

A variety of models of the mental organisation of arithmetical facts has been proposed. One influential view has been that children learn to associate $3 + 5$ with several answers, but the association with 8 will end up as the strongest (Siegler & Shrager, 1984). Another view is that facts are typically stored as specifically verbal associations, though subtraction and division require further processes of "semantic elaboration" involving manipulation of an analogue magnitude representation (Dehaene & Cohen, 1995). In both models, retrieval will depend on the learning history of the individual. Thus, facts that are learned earlier or practiced more will show greater accessibility.

The single strongest argument against these views is that retrieval times show a very strong *problem-size effect* for single-digit problems: the larger the sum or product the longer the problem takes to solve (Ashcraft et al., 1992). This factor is much more potent than how frequently the sum is experienced (see Butterworth et al., 2001).

Note also that children who are using a counting strategy to solve arithmetic problems are not using memory retrieval. It is likely that memories are laid down during Stage 3 of counting on from larger addends. This would mean that the child would work out the result of larger addend + smaller addend (rather than first addend + second addend) and store it in that form. Some evidence for this comes from Butterworth et al. (2001), who showed that adults, who presumably retrieve answers, are quicker to solve Larger Addend + Smaller Addend problems than Smaller Addend + Larger Addend problems. The frequency of the problems in textbooks was not a good predictor of solution times. Both this and the problem-size effect suggest that addition facts are organised in terms of number size rather than as orthogonal a network of associations modulated by practice effects.

Similar results were obtained for children, six to ten years old, doing multiplication. Larger × Smaller was faster than Smaller × Larger even though the (Italian) education system taught Smaller × Larger earlier (Butterworth et al., 2003). For example, 2×6 is in the (Italian) 2× table which is taught before 6×2, which is in the 6× table (Butterworth et al., 2003). In fact, this study showed that children start by privileging the form in which the problem is taught, and later reorganise their memory store to privilege the Larger × Smaller format. Again, this suggests a specifically numerical organisation of arithmetical facts. They are not just rote associations.

Multiplication, division and fractions

Curricula typically introduce multiplication and division later than addition and subtraction, and explain them in terms of repeated addition and repeated subtraction and partitions of sets, thus building on concepts of sets and numerosities. Indeed, Piaget's (1952) treatment of multiplication is in terms of one-to-many correspondence some years later than addition and subtraction. However, ideas of division as sharing occurs very early in development, in some respects earlier even than counting (Nunes & Bryant, 1996), and the idea of a half as the partition of a set, is introduced in Year 1 in the UK (DfEE, 1999). Some multiplication problems can certainly be solved by addition

However, thinking about multiplication or division of two numbers just in terms of sets with one-many correspondences fails to do justice to the kinds of situation the child encounters in everyday life, as well as in the classroom. Prices such as "50p each", is neither the set of objects to be bought, nor the monetary set of the cost. Rather it is a relationship between the two sets, and remains the same (is conserved, if you will) whether six objects are bought or 60. So, multiplication by the price does not increase the price, but only the cost. The price is a ratio, or a kind of division, which is conserved under some types of multiplication. For example, 2/4 is the same ratio as 4/8 or 100/200. Understanding this is fundamental to understanding a whole range of primary school mathematics, including multiplication, division and fractions.

These kinds of numbers are often referred to as "intensive quantities", to distinguish them from numbers whose meanings are "extensive", that is, sets (Schwartz, 1988). Interpreting numbers as intensive quantities is needed for everyday problems involving temperature and concentration. Children of six to eight believe that if you add two cups of water, each at 40°C, the resulting mixture will be warmer than the originals, because you are adding temperatures (Stavy & Tirosh, 2000); and children of ten to 11 find it hard to work out which of two mixtures of orange juice concentrate and water will taste more orangey: three cups of concentrate to two cups of water, or four cups of concentrate to three cups of water (Noelting, 1980a; 1980b). In neither type of case, does a grasp of numerosity fully prepare the child to reason in the appropriate way. Piaget (1952) noted that problems involving proportions would be difficult.

Division also introduces a new type of number in terms of fractions and decimals, namely, rational numbers. These will only have been encountered previously in the concept of a half, but they are important in the everyday context of measures. Again, concepts entailed by numerosities (such as each number has a unique successor) will not work in these contexts.

Nunes & Bryant (1996), in a very useful review, begin their discussion of multiplicative reasoning with the caution: this "is a very complicated topic because it takes different forms and it deals with many situations, and that means that the empirical research on this topic is complicated too" (Nunes & Bryant, 1996, p. 143). It seems clear that where the child can think about multiplication and division as manipulations on sets, then it is relatively easy to acquire, but when the task demands grasp of numbers as intensive quantities then it is difficult.

Understanding arithmetical concepts

Children enter school with informal concepts of number and arithmetic based on their experiences of counting and calculation, however, much educational practice was, and still is, focused on drilling basic arithmetical facts such as number bonds and tables. The theoretical justification came from the work of the American psychologist and educationalist, Edward Thorndike, formulator of the "law of effect" – or what we would now call "reinforcement" – which stated that associations that lead to "satisfying states of affairs" are reinforced, those that lead to unsatisfying states weakened. The idea then was to build networks of reinforced associations between number combinations such as 5 + 3 and their arithmetical result (Thorndike, 1922). As the network, carefully constructed by the teacher, is built in the mind of the child, so the generalisations (concepts and laws) would be grasped. Of course, Thorndike insisted that drilling the facts had to be fun, which meant, among other things, being able to see their practical applications.

More recently, the "distribution of associations" model (Siegler & Shrager, 1984) has been influential. Here it is assumed that the child may associate a number combination with both the wrong and the correct answer. The key to arithmetical success is to strengthen the association with the right answer. The model predicts that the performance on single digit arithmetical fact tasks will be the relative frequency of the association between the problem (e.g. 6 + 3, 6 × 3, 6 − 3, 6 ÷ 3) and the correct solution (9, 18, 3, 2) as compared with the frequency of association between the problem and incorrect solutions.

Even as Thorndike's approach was being taken up by educators, an alternative was being pursued by Brownell, who advocated "meaningful learning" rather than drill (Brownell, 1935). Although research showed that drill can make retrieval of facts faster, transfer of learning to new problems was much better with meaningful learning. The time course of developing an understanding arithmetical concepts and principles, and applying them in a meaningful way, is thus likely to be heavily influenced by the educational practices the child undergoes (Canobi et al., 1998).

Commutativity and associativity

The role of understanding has been tested on commuted pairs of addition facts (6 + 3, 3 + 6) and multiplication facts (6 × 3, 3 × 6).

If commutativity is understood, then is it necessary or even desirable to store in long-term memory both forms of the commute? As we saw above, there is evidence that the form M (larger) + n (smaller) is accessed more readily than n + M (Butterworth et al., 2001). This does not, however, entail understanding. It may just mean that the child has learned that it does not matter in which order the addends appear.

As mentioned above, Butterworth et al. (2003) found that children of six to ten years of age learning multiplication tables reorganise their memories to privilege M × n, over n × M, even when n × M was learned earlier and presumably practiced more. Again, this suggests, though does not prove, that these children understand the commutativity of multiplication.

Interestingly, some cultures do not teach the whole set of multiplication facts from 1 × 1 to 9 × 9 in tabular form. In China, they only teach one half of the set, beginning with 2 × 2 (the 1× table being considered trivial) to 2 × 9; but since 2 × 3 has already been learned, the 3× table begins with 3 × 3, and so on. In this way, only 36 facts have to be acquired, and the equivalence of the commuted pairs has to be learned (Yin Wengang, personal communication). Research shows that Chinese adults are more accurate and quicker at solving multiplication problems than their Western peers (LeFevre & Liu, 1997). Although this has been attributed to more drill (Campbell & Xue, 2001; Penner-Wilger et al., 2002), it may reflect exactly the opposite – fewer facts to memorise and better understanding.

Complementarity

Piaget (1952) has argued, quite reasonably, that a child does not really understand addition or subtraction without understanding the relationship between them. That is, if 5 + 3 equals 8, then 8 − 5 must equal 3, and 8 − 3 must equal 5. This is the principle of complementarity (sometimes called "inverse operations"). All this should follow from an understanding of sets and numerosities: if set B is added to set A, and then removed, the resulting numerosity will still be A.

Do children understand the principle of complementarity, and if so at what age or stage does this understanding begin? Now, of course, it is perfectly possible to arrive at the correct answer without understanding the principle of complementarity. Conversely, it is possible to understand the principle, yet sometimes get the answer wrong. This means that the ability or inability to solve these problems is not a sure guide to understanding. Rather, investigators have asked whether "inversion" problems that can be solved by the principle are solved better than control problems that cannot. Starkey & Gelman (1982) found no convincing evidence for understanding in children of three to five years of age, while other researchers have found evidence of understanding in older children (Stern, 1992).

A systematic study of this issue was reported by Bryant et al. (1999). They looked at five–seven-year-olds, and carefully controlled for types of solution strategies that might be used. For example, in a task using a set of objects, if three new objects are added, and then exactly the same are taken away, then the correct answer may be achieved on the basis of a general "undoing" Principle, that could apply to non-numerical situations such as splashing paint on a wall and washing it off. Bryant et al. controlled for this by comparing adding and removing the same objects, with adding and removing the same number of different objects. They also looked at equivalent problems with numerals. Children were much more successful with inversion problems, such as 12 + 9 − 9, than control problems matched for sum, such as 10 + 10 − 8. What is more, they could use the procedure in more complex problems that required decomposition of the subtrahend. Thus, they appeared to make use of the procedure in problems such as 7 + 4–5 by decomposing

5 into 4 + 1. Indeed, many of the children revealed by analysis of performance to be using the procedure were able to state it in words, but by no means all.

Although the children who used the procedure to solve inversion problems did better overall than those who calculated the solutions, by no means all the children who did well used the principle. Factor analyses and correlations revealed two separate factors: a calculating factor and an understanding factor. Similar issues arise in connection with complementarity of multiplication and division. If $9 \times 3 = 27$ is known, then $27 \div 9 = 3$, and $27 \div 3 = 9$ should both follow without the need for calculation.

Table 5.1 summarises the principal milestones in the normal development of arithmetic.

Table 5.1 Milestones in the early development of arithmetical competence.

Age (year;month)	Milestones (typical study)
0;0	Can discriminate on the basis of small numerosities (Antell & Keating, 1983)
0;4	Can add and subtract one (Wynn, 1992)
0;11	Discriminates increasing from decreasing sequences of numerosities (Brannon, 2002)
2;0	Begins to learn sequence of counting words (Fuson, 1992); can do one-to-one correspondence in a sharing task (Potter & Levy, 1968)
2;6	Recognises that number words mean more than one ("grabber") (Wynn, 1990)
3;0	Counts out small numbers of objects (Wynn, 1990)
3;6	Can add and subtract one with objects and number words (Starkey & Gelman, 1982); Can use cardinal principle to establish numerosity of set (Gelman & Gallistel, 1978)
4;0	Can use fingers to aid adding (Fuson & Kwon, 1992)
5;0	Can add small numbers without being able to count out sum (Starkey & Gelman, 1982)
5;6	Understands commutativity of addition and counts on from larger (Carpenter & Moser, 1982); can count correctly to 40 (Fuson, 1988)
6;0–7;0	"Conserves" number (Piaget, 1952)
6;6	Understands complementarity of addition and subtraction (Bryant et al, 1999); can count correctly to 80 (Fuson, 1988)
7;0	Retrieves some arithmetical facts from memory (LeFevre et al., 1996)

From words to symbols

Typically children will acquire counting words and use them for counting before they learn numerals 1, 2, 3, … This creates a problem. Words in all languages use a *name-value* system. That is, powers of ten are given special names: *ten, hundred, thousand, million*. In English, multiples of ten are given special names: *ten, twenty, thirty, forty* … The numerals, by contrast, use a *place-value* system so that the same symbol means different powers or multiples of ten depending on its position.

Teachers tell me that the transition from name-value to place-value causes difficulty for many children, especially early learners. This has been nicely demonstrated by asking children to write spoken numbers as numerals, and read numerals as spoken numbers by Richard Power and Maria dal Martello of Padua University in Italy. They asked Italian seven-year-olds to write to dictation one-, two-, three-, four-, five- and six-digit numbers. All were completely correct on one- and two-digit numbers, but all made some mistakes for larger numbers. Here are some examples of their "syntactic errors" which confused name and place value.

1.   Cento venti cinque (one hundred and twenty-five) → 10025
2.   Tre mila cento novanta quattro (three thousand one hundred and ninety-four) → 300010094.

This type of error was common. What seems to have happened is that the learners are still in name-value mode for 3-digit numbers and above. So they take "one hundred" as a name to be written, as 100, and "three thousand" as a name written as 3,000. However, at this stage of their numerical development, they do not have a correct understanding of the positional notation of place value, but they do know something. Thus the children above don't write "three thousand" as 31,000. Other children will. Because these children are always correct on two digit numbers, Power and dal Martello conclude there is a different type of rule for constructing them (Power & dal Martello, 1990).

These researchers also looked at children reading the numerals. Again, reading two-digit strings is almost always correct, but reading three-digit and longer strings leads to errors for most children.

Here are examples of the kind of errors for three digit strings the seven-year-olds make.

■   Misplaced "cento"   371 cento tre (hundred three)
■   Consecutive -ty words   834 ottanta trenta quattro (eighty thirty-four)
■   Fragmentation   371 trenta sette e uno (thirty-seven and one)
■   Ignoring part of stimulus   566 cinquanta sei (fifty-six)

Zeros give particular problems with understanding their positional value. Here are two examples of interpreting "0" as meaning thousand instead:

- 609   sessanta mila nove (sixty thousand nine)
- 5604   cinquanta sei mila quattro (fifty-six thousand four)

However, there is little evidence that it is particularly difficult for dyscalculics. Having trouble understanding small numerosities should not really affect these large numbers since they won't be interpreted in terms of sets anyway. The philosopher Bertrand Russell introduced a useful distinction between "knowledge by acquaintance", which would be how we understand numbers in terms of sets of objects which we have encountered, and "knowledge by description". Here we have learned something about numbers from the way in which they have been described in words or in symbols – for example, that "four hundred and three" is bigger than "four hundred and two", or that "403" is bigger than "402" (Russell, 1912).

Learning the words or numerals should be independent of their representation in terms of sets. It turns out that this seems to be the case in the brain. Brain damage can lead to specific problems that mirror those made by early learners, even when calculation is relatively spared. We reported a patient with left parietal damage who was perfect on selecting the larger of two written or spoken numbers up to five digits, and whose spoken calculation was unimpaired, and whose written calculation was poor but not disastrous. However, he made errors with numbers longer than three digits, such as "1000,945" for "One thousand nine hundred and forty five", or "24000,105" for "twenty four thousand one hundred and five". Because he was able to read digits correctly, after two days, he realized that he was writing too many zeros, and thereafter performed correctly (Cipolotti et al., 1994). In an earlier example, from 1933, two US neurologists reported a patient who wrote "10011" for "one hundred and eleven", and for "two thousand five hundred" he wrote "2000500". However, his calculation and number knowledge was severely impaired, and he had difficulty in reading strings of digits (Singer & Low, 1933). More generally, zeros are hard for patients, and a recent study of patients with *right hemisphere lesions* found zero difficulties associated with a brain area called the right insula (Benavides-Varela et al., 2016) (see Chapter 6 for more on the brain).

Summary

- Learning to count and to calculate is based on an innate core capacity for representing the numerosity of sets.
- Based on this sense of numerosity, infants have arithmetical expectations of the effects of adding or taking away set members on the numerosity of the set.

- Learning to count aloud is likely to be the child's first encounter with numerical culture and links existing representations of numerosity with the counting words.
- Counting words use a name value system, and learning to relate name values to place values is an important and sometimes difficult step in becoming numerate in a numerate society,

References

Antell, S. E., & Keating, D. P. (1983). Perception of numerical invariance in neonates. *Child Development, 54*, 695–701.

Ashcraft, M. H., Donley, R., Halas, M. A., & Vakali, M. (1992). Working memory, automaticity and problem difficulty. In J. I. D. Campbell (Ed.), *The Nature and Origins of Mathematical Skills* (Vol. Advances in Psychology, 91, pp. 301–329). Amsterdam: North-Holland.

Benavides-Varela, S., Passarini, L., Butterworth, B., Rolma, G., Burgio, F., Pitteri, M., Meneghello, F., Shallice, T., & Semenza, C. (2016). Zero in the brain: a voxel-based lesion–symptom mapping study in right hemisphere damaged patients. *Cortex, 77*, 38–53.

Brannon, E. M. (2002). The development of ordinal numerical knowledge in infancy. *Cognition, 83*(3), 223–240.

Brownell, W. A. (1935). Psychological Considerations in the Learning and the Teaching of Arithmetic. *The Teaching of Arithmetic*. The tenth yearbook of the National Council of Teachers of Mathematics. New York: Teachers College, Columbia University.

Bryant, P., Christie, C., & Rendu, A. (1999). Children's understanding of the relation between addition and subtraction: Inversion, identity, and decomposition. *Journal of Experimental Child Psychology, 74*, 194–212.

Butterworth, B. (1999). *The Mathematical Brain*. London: Macmillan.

Butterworth, B., Girelli, L., Zorzi, M., & Jonckheere, A. R. (2001). Organisation of addition facts in memory. *Quarterly Journal of Experimental Psychology, 54A*, 1005–1029.

Butterworth, B., Marchesini, N., & Girelli, L. (2003). Organisation of multiplication facts in memory: Developmental trends. In A. Baroody & A. Dowker (Eds), *The Development of Arithmetical Concepts and Skills*. Mahwah, NJ: LEA.

Canobi, Katherine H., Reeve, R., & Pattison, Philippa E. (1998). The Role of Conceptual Understanding in Children's Addition Problem Solving. *Developmental Psychology, 34*(5), 882–891.

Carpenter, T. P., & Moser, J. M. (1982). The development of addition and subtraction problem solving skills. In T. P. Carpenter, J. M. Moser, & T A Romberg (Eds), *Addition and Subtraction: A Cognitive Perspective* (Vol. LEA, pp. 9–24). Hillsdale, NJ.

Cipolotti, L., Butterworth, B., & Warrington, E. K. (1994). From "One thousand nine hundred and forty-five" to 1000,945. *Neuropsychologia, 32*, 503–509.

Dehaene, S., & Cohen, L. (1995). Towards and anatomical and functional model of number processing. *Mathematical Cognition, 1*, 83–120.

DfEE (Department for Education and Employment). (1999). *The National Numeracy Strategy: Framework for Teaching Mathematics from Reception to Year 6*. Sudbury, Suffolk: DfEE Publications.

Fuson, K. C. (1988). *Children's Counting and Concepts of Number*. New York: Springer Verlag.

Fuson, K. C. (1992). Relationships between counting and cardinality from age 2 to 8. In J. Bideaud, C. Meljac, & J. P. Fisher (Eds), *Pathways to Number, Children's Developing Numerical Abilities*. Hillsdale, NJ: LEA.

Fuson, K. C., & Kwon, Y. (1992). Learning addition and subtraction: Effects of number words and other cultural tools. In J. Bideaud, C. Meljac, & J. P. Fisher (Eds), *Pathways to Number, Children's Developing Numerical Abilities*. Hillsdale, NJ: LEA.

Gelman, R., & Gallistel, C. R. (1978). *The Child's Understanding of Number* (1986 ed.). Cambridge, MA: Harvard University Press.

LeFevre, J.-A., & Liu, J. (1997). The role of experience in numerical skill: Multiplication performance in adults from Canada and China. *Mathematical Cognition*, 3, 31–62.

LeFevre, J.-A., Sadesky, G. S., & Bisanz, J. (1996). Selection of procedures in mental addition: Reassessing the problem size effect in adults. *Journal of Experimental Psychology: Learning, Memory, and Cognition*, 22, 216–230.

Noelting, G. (1980a). The development of proportional reasoning and the ratio concept. Part I -Differentiation of stages. *Educational Studies in Mathematics*, 11, 217–253.

Noelting, G. (1980b). The development of proportional reasoning and the ratio concept. Part II Problem-structure at successive stages: problem-solving strategies and the mechanism of adaptive restructuring. *Educational Studies in Mathematics*, 11, 331–363.

Nunes, T., & Bryant, P. (1996). *Children Doing Mathematics*. Oxford: Blackwell.

Penner-Wilger, M., Leth-Steensen, C., & LeFevre, J.-A. (2002). Decomposing the problem-size effect: A comparison of response time distributions across cultures. *Memory & Cognition*, 30, 1160–1167.

Piaget, J. (1952). *The Child's Conception of Number*. London: Routledge & Kegan Paul.

Potter, M. C., & Levy, E. I. (1968). Spatial enumeration without counting. *Child Development*, 39, 265–272.

Power, R. J. D., & dal Martello, M. F. (1990). The dictation of Italian numerals. *Language and Cognitive Processes*, 5, 237–254.

Russell, B. (1912). *The Problems of Philosophy*. Oxford: Oxford University Press.

Schwartz, J. (1988). Intensive quantity and referent transforming arithmetic operations. In J. Hiebert & M. Behr (Eds), *Number Concepts and Operations in the Middle Grades*. Hillsdale, NJ: Erlbaum.

Siegler, R. S., & Shrager, J. (1984). Strategy choices in addition and subtraction: How do children know what to do? In C. Sophian (Ed.), *Origins of Cognitive Skills*. Hillsdale, NJ: Lawrence Erlbaum Associates.

Singer, H., & Low, A. A. (1933). Acalculia (Henschen): A clinical study. *Archives of Neurology & Psychiatry*, 29(3), 467–498. doi: 10.1001/archneurpsyc.1933.02240090037003

Starkey, P., & Gelman, R. (1982). The development of addition and subtraction abilities prior to formal schooling in arithmetic. In T. P. Carpenter, J. M. Moser, & T. A. Romberg (Eds), *Addition and Subtraction: A Cognitive Perspective* (pp. 99–116). Hillsdale, NJ: LEA.

Stavy, R., & Tirosh, D. (2000). *How Students (Mis-)Understand Science and Mathematics*. New York: Teachers College Press.

Stern, E. (1992). Spontaneous use of conceptual mathematical knowledge in elementary-school-children. *Contemporary Educational Psychology*, 17, 266–277.

Thorndike, E. L. (1922). *The Psychology of Arithmetic*. New York: The Macmillan Co.

Wynn, K. (1992). Addition and subtraction by human infants. *Nature*, 358, 749–751.

The dyscalculic brain

LEVEL OF EXPLANATION	MEASURES	EDUCATIONAL CONTEXT
BEHAVIOURAL	Number sense Chapter 2	Society, school and home Chapter 8
COGNITIVE	Starter kit for learning arithmetic Chapter 3 Core deficit as the cause of dyscalculia Chapter 4	Assessment Chapter 9
	Development of arithmetic Chapter 5	Intervention Chapter 10
NEURAL	**Brain structures and functions Chapter 6**	Policy Chapter 11
	GENETIC AND OTHER CAUSES Chapter 7	

To understand the neural basis of dyscalculia, we first have to understand how the typical, non-dyscalculic, brain deals with numerical information and calculation. There is now a great deal of evidence from a variety of sources about this. Before modern neuroimaging, most of the evidence came from neurological patients who had suffered from traumatic brain injury or the effects of disease such as stroke or tumours.

Two things have been clear from these studies is that damage, however caused, to the parietal lobes affects basic numerical processes including estimating numerosities and carrying out familiar calculations. Left and right parietal lobes, though both are involved, act in somewhat different ways. Second, that the frontal lobes are involved whenever a novel calculation or an unfamiliar problem is encountered.

Evidence from the damaged brain

Studies of the effects of brain damage on numerical abilities is at least one hundred years old. A Swedish neurologist, Salomon Henschen, showed in a large series of cases, that if the left parietal lobe was damaged then routine numerical tasks were affected. He also believed that the right hemisphere could take over simple numerical tasks if the left hemisphere was damaged. He was clear that "The cases published show clearly that special [brain] centres exist for calculation, and that they are separated from those of language and music" (Henschen, 1926). He notes that language and number are often impaired together in the patient which suggested to him that their centres are close together in the brain, notably in the left hemisphere.

Number network is distinct in the brain

Henschen came to this view from his cases of patients with preserved abilities to speak and comprehend speech, and still able to read and write words, but who had lost the ability to carry out even simple number tasks. He called this condition, I think for the first time, "akalkulie" or acalculia. He also reported patients who had lost the ability to read words, but could still read numbers. In fact, even in the nineteenth century this condition had been observed by a French neurologist, Dejerine, whose patient M. C. was unable to read aloud words or letters, but was able to read single digits.

We have carried out studies of patients that show patterns similar to those observed by Henschen pointing to the distinctiveness of the number network. See Table 6.1

Modularization of the number network

Even within the number network it is possible to find striking dissociations. Henschen, again with careful pioneering observations, noticed that some patients were able to calculate without being able to read aloud the digits. Modern research has confirmed this, with ability to read and write numbers being spared in some patients who cannot calculate, and, paradoxically, being lost in patients who can (Cappelletti, 2015; Cipolotti & van Harskamp, 2001).

Some patients lose arithmetical facts but retain their understanding of arithmetical concepts and principles (patient BE in Table 6.2); while others may retain some facts but lose their understanding of them (patient JG). There are also cases of losing arithmetical procedures, such as carrying or borrowing in multidigit problems (MT).

Even more striking is the finding that patients can lose some arithmetical operations but not others. You might think that the more difficult operations are more likely to be lost, for example, multiplication and not addition. But this isn't the case, as you can see in Table 6.3.

We'll see below that these results from patients are mirrored to a great extent in neuroimaging results.

Table 6.1 Patients who show dissociations between numerical abilities and other cognitive abilities. Patients CG and DRC have severely impaired numerical abilities but spared language and reasoning. By contrast, the other three patients have spared numerical abilities but severely impaired language. Reasoning seems to be independent of both numerical and language abilities. (STM means short term memory. "X" means largely or completely lost, "√" means largely or completely spared.)

Patient	Maths ability	Language ability	STM	IQ/ reasoning
CG (Cipolotti et al, 1991)	X	√	?√	√
DRC (Warrington, 1982)	X	√	√	√
IH (Cappelletti et al, 2001)	√	X	?√	√
SE (Remond-Besuchet et al, 1999)	√	X	X	X
MRF (Butterworth et al, 1996)	√	X	X	√

Table 6.2 Dissociations among different aspects of numerical ability. "X" means largely or completely lost, "√" means largely or completely spared.

Patient	Signs: +, -, x, +	Facts	Procedures	Conceptual knowledge
Two cases Ferro & Botelho,1980	X	√	√	?√
DRC Warrington, 1982	√	X	√	√
MT Girelli & Delazer, 1996	√	√	X	√
DA Hittmair-Delazer et al,1995	√	X	?√	√
JG Delazer & Benke,1997	√	Multiplication only	X	X
BE Hittmair-Delazer et al, 1994	√	Not multiplication	X	√

Table 6.3 Dissociations in neurological patients among the four arithmetical operations. ("X" means largely or completely lost, "√" means largely or completely spared. "nt" means "not tested".)

Pt	+	-	×	÷
FS van Harskamp & Cipolotti, 2001 selective sparing	X	√	√	nt
MAR Dehaene & Cohen, 1997	√	X	√	X
RG Dagenbach & McCloskey, 1992	X	√	X	nt
BE Hittmair-Delazer et al, 1994	√	√	X	X
JG Delazer & Benke, 1997	X	X	√	X
CB Cipolotti & De Lacy Costello, 1995	√	√	√	X

Evidence from neuroimaging

Neuroimaging enables us to get a sense of how these brain regions operate when carrying out a variety of numerical tasks, and also how they are linked together. There is now a wide variety of neuroimaging methods, including fMRI (functional magnetic resonance imaging) that measures regional activations indirectly through tracking how oxygenated blood flows into the activated regions. This means there is a delay between the activation and the measurement which can be as much as six seconds. For faster responses, there is EEG (electroencephalography) which can measure changes in the brain's electrical activity almost instantaneously, but at the price of much poorer localization than fMRI, and it is usually hard to get information in the deeper layers of the brain. One method that can combine fast response and reasonable localization is MEG (magnetoencephalography) which measures changes in the magnetic fields of the brain induced by activity in the neurons. There are other methods that I will mention briefly below as I come to them.

MRI (magnetic resonance imaging) also allows us to explore another aspects of the neural circuitry: the *structure* of the *grey matter* – the neuron cell bodies responsible for the activity, and also the *white matter* fibres that connect one cell to another.

This isn't the place to go into how these methods work. There are many good accounts available for the interested reader (see in the references). However, all these methods depend on one key logical inference: comparison.

Thus, to know whether the *structure* of dyscalculic brains is different from typical brains, then of course we need to know the structure of typical brains. This is more difficult than it seems since all brains are different one from another in various ways – size, weight, arrangement of the lobes and sulci (grooves). This means that it will take something like the average of a number of typical brains mapped onto to a standardized brain template, in comparison with the average of a number of dyscalculic brains.

To know whether a brain region is active during a particular numerical task, one needs to compare the task activations with activations for something else. I'll give examples as we go along. To know whether dyscalculic brains activate differently, we need to compare them with typical brains doing the same task. Again, each of our brains will activate somewhat differently doing the same task because our brains are structured a bit differently, and the brain's history of doing the task will be different (for example, did we learn the multiplication tables through rote repetition of all 81 pairs of numbers, or in some other way; and how much did we practice and how well did we link table knowledge to other aspects of mathematics). This means that we need to take averages of task activations from several people.

Now there have been many studies that show that two regions of the brain are reliably active for almost any numerical task – comparing numbers, comparing the numerosity of sets, carrying out simple calculation. These areas – the *intraparietal sulci* (plural of *sulcus*) are related to *number abstraction* – that is, these regions respond whether the numbers are presented as arrays of dots, or digits, or number words. In particular, there is evidence that one function of these regions is to extract numerosities from the environment. Even if the brain has had no experience of numerals or counting words, these regions respond to numerosities in a systematic way, so the homologous regions in monkey brains respond to numerosities just as our brains do; not only that, but the links between the parietal and frontal lobes is similar too (Nieder, 2005).

The arithmetical brain

Now, many studies have identified the same network of regions in the brain for carrying our arithmetical tasks. It is important to bear in mind that all studies of brain activation are essentially comparisons, either between several tasks or between two or more groups of people. You need to compare tasks otherwise you cannot separate out the brain activities you are interested in from other brain activities you are not interested in.

One of the first studies to identify the arithmetic network compared two arithmetical tasks with simply reading numbers, so it was able separate out calculation activity from what happens when you see numbers. In fact, the study by a French team used two arithmetical tasks: retrieving a solution from memory, for example, the solution to 6×4, and carrying out a more complex and demanding calculation, 37×14 (see Figure 6.1).

A team from the Catholic University of Louvain in Belgium led by Mauro Pesenti, replicated this result using a slightly different comparison task, and a different calculation task (see Figure 6.2).

Now the parietal and frontal regions work together when carrying out arithmetical tasks. It was subsequently established that one additional area on the

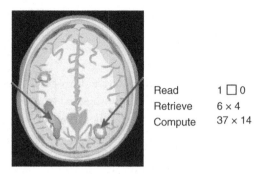

Read   1 □ 0
Retrieve   6 × 4
Compute   37 × 14

Figure 6.1 The arithmetical network in the adult brain looking down on the brain. The tasks to be performed are on the right of the brain picture. See text for further explanation.

From Zago et al., 2001.

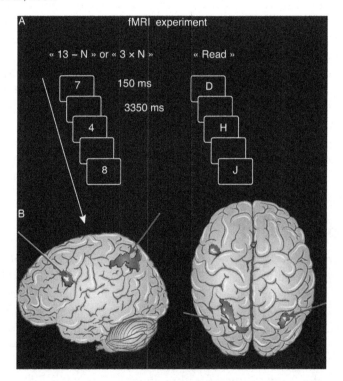

Figure 6.2 The arithmetic network. The arithmetic tasks are subtraction and multiplication. Adult participants were instructed to subtract mentally the presented digit from 11 or 13, or to multiply it by 3 or 4, and to provide the response verbally. Instructions emphasized both speed and accuracy. After subtracting the activations from the reading tasks, the activations for the calculations (in red and orange) are shown in side view and top view. This network corresponds very closely with the network in Figure 6.1, suggesting a stable network that supports subtraction, addition, multiplication retrieval and complex calculation. The critical regions are in the intraparietal sulci (arrows) in both left and right hemispheres.

From Andres et al., 2011.

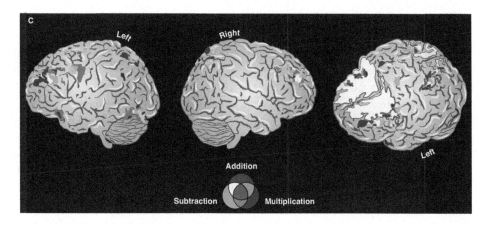

Figure 6.3 Neuroimaging reveals distinct activations, as well as common ones, for the three of the four arithmetical operations.

From Arsalidou & Taylor, 2011.

border of the left parietal lobe – the *left angular gyrus* – is more active during trials depending on simple fact retrieval, while the frontal lobes are relatively more active when arithmetical strategies are required (Grabner et al., 2009).

The implication is that the brain comes equipped with a network of regions dedicated to numerical processes. Not only that, but when some individual becomes really good at mathematics, such as expert calculators or professional mathematicians, the same regions are activated (Amalric & Dehaene, 2016; Aydin et al., 2007; Pesenti et al., 2001). Of course, becoming expert involves learning, a lot of learning.

Modularization

We saw from studies of neurological patients that arithmetical operations seem to be independently represented in the brain. A meta-analysis of the neuroimaging results confirms this separation in the brain, despite some common areas (red blobs in Figure 6.3), nevertheless all the activations are in the fronto-parietal network we saw in Figures 6.1 and 6.2.

Very recently, recordings and stimulation directly on the surface of the brain in patients with intractable epilepsy show very specific localization for visual numerals in the inferior temporal gyrus (Daitch et al., 2016; Shum et al., 2013); and for different arithmetical operations (Daitch et al., 2016; Della Puppa et al., 2013; Semenza et al., 2017; Shum et al., 2013).

Numerosity processing

Now this is the network for arithmetic, but how does it relate to representing numerosities? The first study to show that the *intraparietal sulcus bilaterally* (arrowed regions in Figure 6.2) is implicated in this was carried out by one of the major figures in our understanding the brain network for mathematics, the pioneering French neuroscientist,

Stanislas Dehaene and his team. In a review of several studies, they found that the *intraparietal sulcus bilaterally* was activated in almost all numerical tasks. For "number sense" (see Chapter 2) tasks, they found that activation increased as the similarity increased in the number of dots in the sets to be compared. This is called the *distance effect*. In purely behavioural studies, the time to select the set increases as similarity between the two sets increases. This is also true when selecting the larger of two digits: 4 or 5 takes longer to judge than 4 or 8, or two words four or five and four or eight. In fact, one review found that activation in the intraparietal sulcus bilaterally increased in the same way and in the same location in the brain not only for comparing the number of dots, but also for digit and word comparisons (Dehaene et al., 2003).

The *intraparietal sulcus* responds not only to numerosity when the set of dots is presented *simultaneously* – for example in two panels on the screen – but also sequentially. We carried out an experiment in which participants had to judge whether there were more green squares or more red squares when these were presented as a sequence of 30 squares (Piazza et al., 2006) (see Figure 6.4).

One problem with these studies, including the studies with words and digits, is whether the brain is making a decision on the *number* or the *quantity* (which could be a continuous amount). That is, is it making a judgment on the basis of *how many* or just on *how much?* In Chapter 3, I described briefly an alternative to the

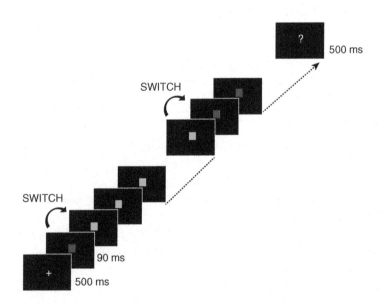

Figure 6.4 Participants were asked to judge at the end of the sequence ("?") whether there were more red or more green squares. In the auditory condition, there was an equivalent sequence of high and low tones requiring a judgment of more high or more low. The same brain areas - intraparietal sulcus bilaterally – was activated in both tasks suggesting there is a region that supports "number abstraction".

From Piazza et al., 2006.

view presented in this book in which numerical magnitudes are represented in the brain not by representations of sets but by analogue magnitudes – the "Analogue Magnitude System" due originally to Dehaene. We set out to test which of us was correct with my colleagues at the Institute of Cognitive Neuroscience at UCL, Fulvia Castelli and Daniel Glaser. In this study, we had four separate tasks that participants carried out while lying in the scanner (see Figure 6.5).

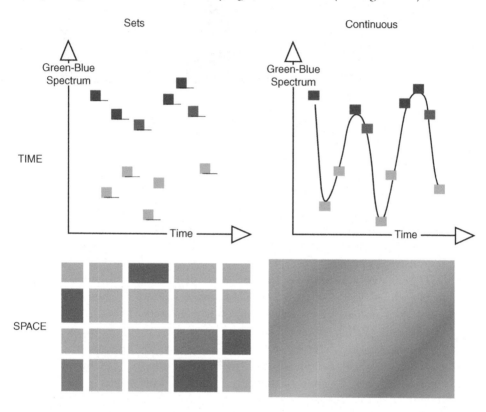

Figure 6.5 For this study, we had two questions: are there regions specific to processing the numerosity of sets and not just to how much stuff is perceived? And, will these regions respond to numerosity abstractly – in this case, independently of how the sets are presented? The top view of the brain (the slice just above the ears) on the left shows two small regions in the IPS (intraparietal sulcus) where the activation depended on the ratio of blue to green in both the Time and the Space tasks. In the Space task example, there are 6 blues to 14 greens, and is an easy decision; 9 blues to 11 greens would be more difficult. The activations here – and nowhere else in the brain – were proportional to the ratios of blue to green. These two regions in the intraparietal sulci bilaterally (indicated by white blobs in the left-hand brain picture below) are activated by the abstract numerosity of the sets, that is irrespective of mode of presentation. The two regions identified in Castelli et al. (2006) are the white blobs. Here they are superimposed on the yellow blobs of the arithmetic network (copied from Figure 6.2 above, Andres et al., 2011). (*continued overleaf*)

From Castelli et al., 2000.

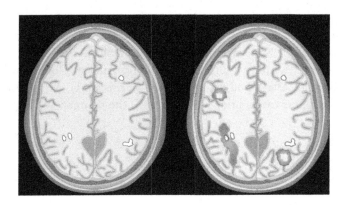

Figure 6.5 (*Continued*)

The learning brain

The structure of brain regions and their connections change in response to experiences, including learning. This is called "brain plasticity". In fact, the same cognitive task may recruit changes in the current network, or even a different network, in response to experience.

There's a good example of this in a study of adults learning new multiplication facts such as 17 × 4. As we saw in Figures 6.1 and 6.2, the *arithmetical network* involves the *intraparietal sulci bilaterally* connected to the *frontal lobe*, mainly the left frontal lobe. When we are confronted by a new problem we engage the *frontal lobes* - the region where we set up tasks, define goals, and assess whether a goal has been achieved. So, for most of us, 17 × 4 is a new problem and will engage the frontal lobes. By contrast, when we retrieve a known fact, such as 7 × 4 = 28, then the frontal lobes are only minimally involved. We also know that arithmetical fact retrieval depends on the parietal lobe, actually on a region just below the IPS called the *angular gyrus*. This predicts that learning will involve a shift from a network with a lot of frontal activation to a network with mainly parietal activation. This is exactly what my friends in Innsbruck, Margarete Delazer and Anja Ischebeck and their colleagues, established (see Figure 6.6).

As I mentioned, real experts activate the same network (and sometimes additional regions, depending on the task), and it turns out that the amount of practice affects brain structure so that the longer a professional mathematician has been practicing his or her trade in a university, the greater the grey matter density in the left parietal lobe (Aydin et al., 2007).

Brain development

As well as changing as a result of learning, the brain changes with age and maturation. For example, the peak volume of grey matter in the frontal lobes is at about 13 years

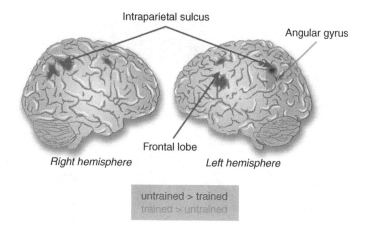

Figure 6.6 The effect of training with new multiplication facts, such as 17x4. When new, these problems involved frontal lobe activation; after training, the activation was in the angular gyrus. Thus learning a new arithmetical fact changes the pattern of activation in carrying out the task.

From Ischebeck et al., 2006.

in boys and 11 years in girls, and then volume reduces from about 14 years. There's a similar trajectory in the parietal lobe, but with the peaks a year or so earlier.

Number sense

The neural basis for number sense also changes. As we have seen, in adults the IPS in both hemispheres is almost always involved in any numerical task. Daniel Ansari and Bibek Dhital used a very simple non-symbolic numerosity comparison task that we have seen before (Figure 6.7) with children aged around ten years and adults aged 20 years.

Elizabeth Brannon and her team at Duke University who, extraordinarily, explore the neural basis of numerical abilities in two very difficult participants – human babies and monkeys. Here, they turn their attention to the more tractable problem of the neural networks activated in children of six to seven years and in adults. In children, the activation is more or less equally balanced between hemispheres, but in the adult, there is more activation in the left (see Figure 6.8).

Arithmetic: the frontal to parietal shift

There is also a developmental shift from frontal lobes in children to parietal in young adults in carrying out simple a + b = c type calculation (Rivera et al., 2005) In fact, it is possible to see this in the strategies children use. As I noted in Chapter 3, children progress from effortful counting strategies to less demanding retrieval. So in the early stages of development, a child will solve 3 + 5 = ? By "counting all" – that is, counting (some will use their fingers to do this) *one, two, three* pause *four, five, six, seven, eight*. A later and more sophisticated strategy that requires understanding that 3 + 5 = 5 + 3, would start with five, and continue *six,*

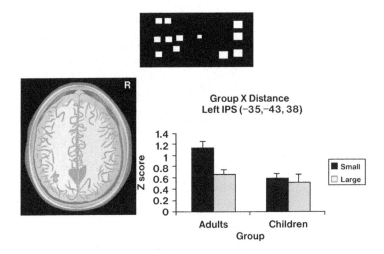

Figure 6.7 Children and adults had to select the side with the most squares (Top panel shows an example of the stimuli). The task is easy when difference in the number of square is large – e.g. seven squares vs four – and difficult when the difference is small. This is known as "the distance effect". Both adults and children show a distance effect in the left IPS, but there are two age-related changes: the effect is greater in adults (bar chart). Adults activate the left IPS more than the right, whereas children the activation is similar in both hemispheres: the difference is depicted by the red area in the brain image.

From Ansari & Dhital, 2006.

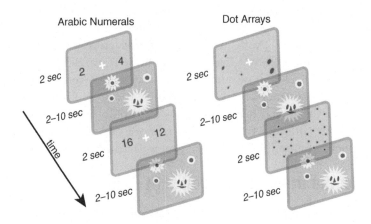

Figure 6.8 Children (six to seven years) and adults doing the same simple numerical tasks: selecting the larger of the two numbers and selecting the more numerous of the dot arrays. In children, the activation (in red) is roughly equal in the two hemispheres, while in the adult there is more activation in the left hemisphere (in green).

From Cantlon et al., 2009.

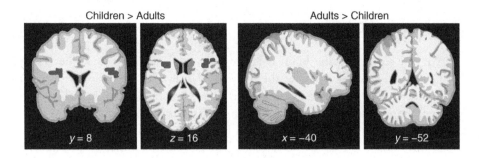

Figure 6.8 (*Continued*)

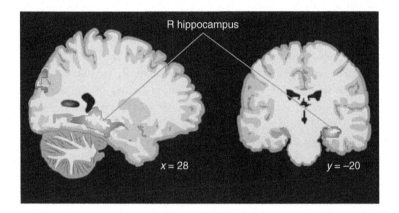

Figure 6.9 Children (seven to nine years) who retrieve answers to single digit addition problems, such as 3 + 5 = ?, use the general memory system of the hippocampus more than children who still use counting to solve these problems.

From Cho et al., 2012.

seven, eight. This is sometimes called the "Min strategy" or "Counting on from smaller", because you only count the smaller number. There comes a point when the child simply remembers that both 3 + 5 and 5 + 3 add up to 8, and therefore only needs to *retrieve* the solution. In fascinating experiment, a very influential team at Stanford University in California, led by Vinod Menon, found that children seven to nine years who used retrieval showed more activation than the counters in the brain region associated with memory, namely the hippocampus (Cho et al., 2012) (see Figure 6.8). There was also more activation in prefrontal cortex, which is where we set up tasks, define goals, and assess whether a goal has been achieved, including the whole process of looking for a memory and checking that we have found it. The other interesting finding was that the re-trievers also showed more activation in the *angular gyrus* which we have seen is associated with arithmetical fact retrieval, but whereas in adults retrieval seems confined to the left angular gyrus, here the activations are in both the left and right angular gyrus.

The dyscalculic brain

We can see where the brain is active when it's carrying out numerical tasks, so now it's time to ask whether the brains of dyscalculics are different in structure or functioning in just the regions supporting arithmetic. In particular, if the *core deficit* hypothesis is correct, there will be abnormalities in the brain regions responsible for numerosity processing in the IPS bilaterally. As I have mentioned many times in this book, there are lots of reasons why an individual may be bad at arithmetic, so it remains possible that people who are very poor at arithmetic, and even dyscalculic according to my definition, have neural differences in other parts of the arithmetic network.

One problem with the available, and still rather limited, research on the dyscalculic brain is the widespread problem of which individuals are classified as dyscalculic. Not all have been tested for a core deficit, and not all are equally bad at arithmetic. Some learners would normally be classed as normal. For example, one study took children who were below 90 on a standardized maths test, which is within one standard deviation of the population mean (Ashkenazi et al., 2012)!

Unsurprisingly, there are wide differences, and even contradictions, in the findings. Some show decreased grey or white matter, others increased; some show decreased activations, others increased. The matter is not helped by studies using different ages, since as we have seen, the key regions change with age. A good general review of the relationship between brain development and arithmetic can be found in (Peters & De Smedt, 2017).

I've tried below to focus on those studies in which either arithmetic performance is in the range predicted by the best prevalence estimates (lowest 4–7%) or where there is a test of the core deficit.

Grey matter structure

The pioneering and classic study of the different *structure* of the dyscalculic brain was carried out by my colleague Elizabeth Isaacs and her team at UCL's Institute of Child Health. They were interested in preterm children with very low birth weight and selected two groups of 12 adolescents each whom they had followed from birth. Both groups had IQs in the normal range, and showed typical cognitive development in other respects, but the dyscalculic group were significantly worse on a standard test of simple arithmetic (called Numerical Operations from the Wechsler Objective Numeric Dimensions battery (Wechsler, 1996)). The brain of each participant was scanned using MRI and the differences in *structure* analysed. The only region in which the two groups differed was in the left intraparietal sulcus, exactly the region we know is involved in basic numerical processing. What is more, this small region turns out to have lower grey matter density in the dyscalculic brain (see Figure 6.10).

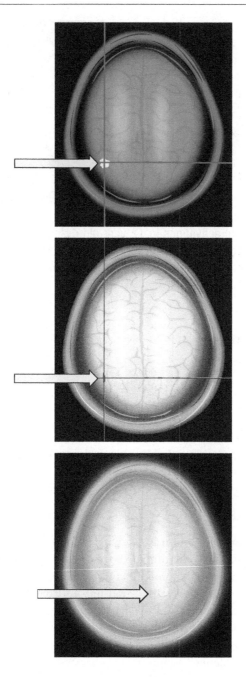

Figure 6.10 The abnormal grey matter in the intraparietal sulci of dyscalculics compared with carefully-matched controls. (A) Left intraparietal sulcus of adolescent dyscalculics (Isaacs et al., 2001). (B) Left intraparietal sulcus of adolescent dyscalculics (Ranpura et al., in preparation). (C) Right intraparietal sulcus of nine-year-old dyscalculics (Rotzer et al., 2008)

From Isaacs et al., 2001.

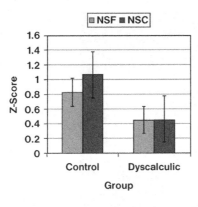
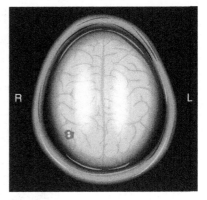

Figure 6.11 Abnormal activations in 12-year-old dyscalculics compared with matched controls in a numerosity comparison task. Notice the absence of a "distance effect" in the dyscalculics. NSF means non-symbolic far; NSC means non-symbolic close. (Right "R" is on the left).

From Price et al., 2007.

Patterns of activation

There is also evidence that this key region activates differently in dyscalculics. A study by (Price et al., 2007) revealed less activation in this region (perhaps in part because of less grey matter) and that it is less sensitive to the distance effect when comparing two sets of squares (using stimuli similar to those in Figure 6.7) (see Figure 6.11). Typically, there is more activation when the distance is small – and the discrimination is more difficult – than when it is large and the discrimination is easier. These dyscalculics showed no effect.

White matter tracts

As we saw in Figures 6.1 and 6.2, carrying out arithmetical tasks – as opposed to simple number tasks, such as number comparison – involves a network of regions. These regions work together and are connected together by longer fibre tracts of *white matter*. These are the *axons* that transmit information from one neuron body (the grey matter) to another. This means that another potential source of difference between dyscalculics and typically developing learners is in this white matter. Are the neurons less well connected in dyscalculics?

There is some evidence to support this, especially the bundle of fibres connecting the parietal to the frontal lobes which are smaller in volume in dyscalculic children than in matched controls (Rykhlevskaia et al., 2009). One problem with this study is that the children (aged eight to nine years) classified as dyscalculic, were not really dyscalculic. On standardized arithmetic tests, Numerical Operations and Mathematical Reasoning (the same tests used by Isaacs et al., 2001) they scored 89 and 103 respectively, where the mean is 100, and one standard deviation is 15. This means they are within the normal range on this test. Admittedly, they were significantly worse than the control group. There were no tests for a deficit in number sense (as described in Chapters 2 and 3). However, reduced white matter volume has been observed in dyscalculic nine-year-olds in the left frontal lobes (Rotzer et al., 2008).

In general, there seems to be a relationship between white matter volume in the tracts that connect parietal to frontal lobes in teenagers but this analysis did not specifically look at dyscalculic learners (Matejko & Ansari, 2015). We found differences in white matter in a small group of dyscalculics – defined by a significant discrepancy between their Numerical Operations score and their full-scale IQ; plus, they were significantly slower on timed simple arithmetic than matched controls, and, critically, significantly slower on *dot enumeration*, the criterion for a *core deficit* in number sense. We also discovered something else interesting – an age trend. The volume of many of the white matter bundles increased with age in the typically-developing controls, but not in the dyscalculics (Ranpura et al., 2013).

Although there is not yet much evidence, the main white matter tracts associated with numerical abilities seem to be those that link the parietal lobes to the frontal lobes – such as the inferior longitudinal fasciculus and the superior longitudinal fasciculus. One other area is implicated – the corpus callosum, especially the posterior part, that links together the right and left parietal lobes (Matejko & Ansari, 2015).

Clearly, there is still much work to be done on how the different parts of the network are connected and how they work together, or do not.

Summary

- Arithmetic processes engage a network comprising the left and right parietal and the left frontal lobes.
- The parietal lobes are engaged during numerosity processing, such as deciding which display has more objects.
- The balance of functioning between the hemispheres changes with age, going from right hemisphere dominance to left hemisphere dominance by adolescence.
- The dyscalculic brain shows abnormalities of structure and activation in the parietal lobes.

References

Amalric, M., & Dehaene, S. (2016). Origins of the brain networks for advanced mathematics in expert mathematicians. *Proceedings of the National Academy of Sciences*, 113(18), 4909–4917. doi: 10.1073/pnas.1603205113

Andres, M., Pelgrims, B., Michaux, N., Olivier, E., & Pesenti, M. (2011). Role of distinct parietal areas in arithmetic: An fMRI-guided TMS study. *NeuroImage*, 54(4), 3048–3056. doi: 10.1016/j.neuroimage.2010.11.009

Ansari, D., & Dhital, B. (2006). Age-related changes in the activation of the intraparietal sulcus during nonsymbolic magnitude processing: An event-related functional magnetic resonance imaging study. *Journal of Cognitive Neuroscience*, 18, 1820–1828.

Arsalidou, M., & Taylor, M. J. (2011). Is 2+2=4? Meta-analyses of brain areas needed for numbers and calculations. *NeuroImage*, 54(3), 2382–2393. doi: 10.1016/j.neuro image.2010.10.009

Ashkenazi, S., Rosenberg-Lee, M., Tenison, C., & Menon, V. (2012). Weak task-related modulation and stimulus representations during arithmetic problem solving in children with developmental dyscalculia. *Developmental Cognitive Neuroscience*, 2, S152–S166. doi: 10.1016/j.dcn.2011.09.006

Aydin, K., Ucar, A., Oguz, K. K., Okur, O. O., Agayev, A., Unal, Z., … Ozturk, S. (2007). Increased gray matter density in the parietal cortex of mathematicians: A Voxel-Based Morphometry study. *American Journal of Neuroradiology*, 28, 1859–1864.

Butterworth, B., Cipolotti, L., & Warrington, E. K. (1996). Short-term memory impairments and arithmetical ability. *Quarterly Journal of Experimental Psychology*, 49A, 251–262.

Cantlon, J. F., Libertus, M. E., Pinel, P., Dehaene, S., Brannon, E. M., & Pelphrey, K. A. (2009). The Neural Development of an Abstract Concept of Number. *Journal of Cognitive Neuroscience*, 21(11), 2217–2229. doi: 10.1162/jocn.2008.21159

Cappelletti, M. (2015). The neuropsychology of acquired number and calculation disorders. In R. Cohen Kadosh & A. Dowker (Eds), *Oxford Handbook of Numerical Cognition* (pp. 808–836). Oxford: OUP.

Cappelletti, M., Butterworth, B., & Kopelman, M. (2001). Spared numerical abilities in a case of semantic dementia. *Neuropsychologia*, 39, 1224–1239.

Castelli, F., Glaser, D. E., & Butterworth, B. (2006). Discrete and analogue quantity processing in the parietal lobe: A functional MRI study. *Proceedings of the National Academy of Sciences of the United States of America*, 103(12), 4693–4698.

Cho, S., Metcalfe, A. W. S., Young, C. B., Ryali, S., Geary, D. C., & Menon, V. (2012). Hippocampal–Prefrontal Engagement and Dynamic Causal Interactions in the Maturation of Children's Fact Retrieval. *Journal of Cognitive Neuroscience*, 24(9), 1849–1866. doi: 10.1162/jocn_a_00246

Cipolotti, L., & Costello, A. d. L. (1995). Selective impairment for simple division. *Cortex*, 31, 433–449.

Cipolotti, L., & van Harskamp, N. (2001). Disturbances of number processing and calculation. In R. S. Berndt (Ed.), *Handbook of Neuropsychology* (2nd ed., Vol. 3, pp. 305–334). Amsterdam: Elsevier Science.

Cipolotti, L., Butterworth, B., & Denes, G. (1991). A specific deficit for numbers in a case of dense acalculia. *Brain*, 114, 2619–2637.

Dagenbach, D., & McCloskey, M. (1992). The organization of arithmetic facts in memory: Evidence from a brain-damaged patient. *Brain and Cognition*, 20(2), 345–366. doi: 10.1016/0278–2626(92)90026–I

Daitch, A. L., Foster, B. L., Schrouff, J., Rangarajan, V., Kaşikçi, I., Gattas, S., & Parvizi, J. (2016). Mapping human temporal and parietal neuronal population activity and functional coupling during mathematical cognition. *Proceedings of the National Academy of Sciences*, 113(46), E7277–E7286. doi: 10.1073/pnas.1608434113

Dehaene, S., & Cohen, L. (1997). Cerebral pathways for calculation: Double dissociation between rote verbal and quantitative knowledge of arithmetic. *Cortex*, 33(2), 219–250.

Dehaene, S., Piazza, M., Pinel, P., & Cohen, L. (2003). Three parietal circuits for number processing. *Cognitive Neuropsychology*, 20, 487–506.

Delazer, M., & Butterworth, B. (1997). A dissociation of number meanings. *Cognitive Neuropsychology*, 14, 613–636.

Della Puppa, A., De Pellegrin, S., d'Avella, E., Gioffrè, G., Munari, M., Saladini, M., … Semenza, C. (2013). Right parietal cortex and calculation processing: intraoperative functional mapping of multiplication and addition in patients affected by a brain tumor. *Journal of Neurosurgery*, 119(5), 1107–1111. doi: 10.3171/2013.6.JNS122445

Ferro, J. M., & Botelho, M. H. (1980). Alexia for arithmetical signs: A cause for disturbed calculation. *Cortex*, 16, 175–180.

Girelli, L., & Delazer, M. (1996). Subtraction bugs in an acalculic patient. *Cortex*, 32, 547–555.

Grabner, R. H., Ansari, D., Koschutnig, K., Reishofer, G., Ebner, F., & Neuper, C. (2009). To retrieve or to calculate? Left angular gyrus mediates the retrieval of arithmetic facts during problem solving. *Neuropsychologia*, 47(2), 604–608.

Henschen, S. E. (1926). On the function of the right hemisphere of the brain in relation to the left in speech, music and calculation. *Brain*, 49(1), 110–123. doi: 10.1093/brain/49.1.110

Hittmair-Delazer, M., Sailer, U., & Benke, T. (1995). Impaired arithmetic facts but intact conceptual knowledge - a single-case study of dyscalculia. *Cortex*, 31, 139–147.

Hittmair-Delazer, M., Semenza, C., & Denes, G. (1994). Concepts and facts in calculation. *Brain*, 117, 715–728.

Isaacs, E. B., Edmonds, C. J., Lucas, A., & Gadian, D. G. (2001). Calculation difficulties in children of very low birthweight: A neural correlate. *Brain*, 124, 1701–1707.

Ischebeck, A., Zamarian, L., Siedentopf, C., Koppelstatter, F., Benke, T., Felber, S., & Delazer, M. (2006). How specifically do we learn? Imaging the learning of multiplication and subtraction. *NeuroImage*, 30(4), 1365–1375.

Matejko, A. A., & Ansari, D. (2015). Drawing connections between white matter and numerical and mathematical cognition: A literature review. Neuroscience & *Biobehavioral Reviews*, 48, 35–52. doi: 10.1016/j.neubiorev.2014.11.006

Nieder, A. (2005). Counting on neurons: The neurobiology of numerical competence. *Nature Reviews Neuroscience*, 6(3), 1–14.

Pesenti, M., Zago, L., Crivello, F., Mellet, E., Samson, D., Duroux, B., … Tzourio-Mazoyer, N. (2001). Mental calculation expertise in a prodigy is sustained by right prefrontal and medial-temporal areas. *Nature Neuroscience*, 4(1), 103–107.

Peters, L., & De Smedt, B. (2017). Arithmetic in the developing brain: A review of brain imaging studies. *Developmental Cognitive Neuroscience*. doi: 10.1016/j.dcn.2017.05.002

Piazza, M., Mechelli, A., Price, C. J., & Butterworth, B. (2006). Exact and approximate judgements of visual and auditory numerosity: An fMRI study. *Brain Research*, 1106, 177–188.

Price, G. R., Holloway, I., Räsänen, P., Vesterinen, M., & Ansari, D. (2007). Impaired parietal magnitude processing in developmental dyscalculia. *Current Biology*, 17(24), R1042–R1043.

Ranpura, A., Isaacs, E., Edmonds, C., Rogers, M., Lanigan, J., Singhal, A., … Butterworth, B. (2013). Developmental trajectories of grey and white matter in dyscalculia. *Trends in Neuroscience and Education*, 2(2), 56–64. doi: 10.1016/j.tine.2013.06.007

Remond-Besuchet, C., Noël, M.-P., Seron, X., Thioux, M., Brun, M., & Aspe, X. (1999). Selective preservation of exceptional arithmetical knowledge in a demented patient. *Mathematical Cognition*, 5, 41–63.

Rivera, S. M., Reiss, S. M., Eckert, M. A., & Menon, V. (2005). Developmental Changes in Mental Arithmetic: Evidence for Increased Functional Specialization in the Left Inferior Parietal Cortex. *Cerebral Cortex*, 15, 1779–1790.

Rotzer, S., Kucian, K., Martin, E., von Aster, M., Klaver, P., & Loenneker, T. (2008). Optimized voxel-based morphometry in children with developmental dyscalculia. *NeuroImage*, 39(1), 417–422.

Rykhlevskaia, E., Uddin, L. Q., Kondos, L., & Menon, V. (2009). Neuroanatomical correlates of developmental dyscalculia: combined evidence from morphometry and tractography. *Frontiers in Human Neuroscience*, 3(51), 1–13. doi: 10.3389/neuro.09.051.2009

Semenza, C., Salillas, E., Di Pellegrin, S., & Della Puppa, A. (2017). Balancing the 2 Hemispheres in Simple Calculation: Evidence From Direct Cortical Electrostimulation. *Cerebral Cortex*, 27(10), 4806–4814. doi: 10.1093/cercor/bhw277

Shum, J., Hermes, D., Foster, B., Dastjerdi, M., Rangarajan, V., Winawer, J., … Parvizi, J. (2013). A brain area for visual numerals. *Journal of Neuroscience*, 33(16), 6709–6715. doi: 10.1523/JNEUROSCI.4558-12.2013

van Harskamp, N. J., & Cipolotti, L. (2001). Selective impairments for addition, subtraction and multiplication. Implications for the organisation of arithmetical facts. *Cortex*, 37, 363–388.

Warrington, E. K. (1982). The fractionation of arithmetical skills: A single case study. *Quarterly Journal of Experimental Psychology*, 34A, 31–51.

Wechsler, D. (1996). *Wechsler Objective Numerical Dimensions* (WOND). London: The Psychological Corporation.

Zago, L., Pesenti, M., Mellet, E., Crivello, F., Mazoyer, B., & Tzourio-Mazoyer, N. (2001). Neural correlates of simple and complex mental calculation. *NeuroImage*, 13(2), 314–327.

7

Heritability and the effects of brain damage on numerical abilities

LEVEL OF EXPLANATION	MEASURES	EDUCATIONAL CONTEXT
BEHAVIOURAL	Number sense Chapter 2	Society, school and home Chapter 8
COGNITIVE	Starter kit for learning arithmetic Chapter 3 Core deficit as the cause of dyscalculia Chapter 4	Assessment Chapter 9
	Development of arithmetic Chapter 5	Intervention Chapter 10
NEURAL	Brain structures and functions Chapter 6	Policy Chapter 11
GENETIC AND OTHER CAUSES Chapter 7		

For most people dyscalculia is congenital: that is, they are born with the condition. For some, brain damage after birth is the cause, and I deal with these individuals later in this chapter.

To say that one is born with this condition does not mean that it is necessarily inherited, nor that it is unchanging. We know this from several sources: from studies of twins, from family studies and from genetic anomalies. That is, it can be *heritable*.

We also know that environmental conditions *before* birth can affect the development of the relevant brain regions. I'll discuss some of these, including prematurity and foetal alcohol syndrome.

Brain damage after birth, often long after birth, can result in dyscalculia, but that its pattern is much more variable than the genetic. This was briefly mentioned in Chapter 6 on the dyscalculic brain.

I'll deal with each of these causes in this chapter.

It is also worth bearing in mind genetic and environmental conditions can affect each other. Environment can trigger or suppress the expression of genes – that is, to simplify, the proteins that are the gene product. Genes may also create a risk factor which in some environments can cause a cognitive abnormality, including dyscalculia, and in others, not; however, these mechanisms have not been extensively explored. Our estimates of heritability will depend on the homogeneity of the environment: so, where people all experience very similar environments – for example, similar educations – then individual genetic differences will appear more pronounced.

Heritability

Twin studies

Box 7.1 What heritability means in twin studies

Twins are two offspring of the same pregnancy. Twins can be either monozygotic ("identical"), meaning that they develop from one zygote, which splits and forms two embryos, and therefore they share exactly the same genes, and are therefore always of the same sex; or dizygotic ("fraternal"), meaning that they develop from two different eggs. In fraternal twins, each twin is fertilized by its own sperm cell, and share on average 50% of their genes, the same as between any siblings, and the twins can be of different sexes.

The logic of twin studies is essentially simple: are identical twins more similar to each other on the trait of interest (the phenotype) than fraternal twins. To estimate the degree of heritability of a trait of interest (the phenotype), such as numerical ability or dyscalculia, we ask whether monozygotic twins are more similar (the technical term is "concordant") than the dizygotic twins. Of course, twins usually share a common upbringing and environment though not an identical upbringing, for example, if one of them gets sick and the other does not.

Now, even concordant twins are not wholly concordant. That is, they are not identical on the trait of interest. The difference between the phenotypes of a pair of monozygotic twins is assumed to be due to a non-shared environmental circumstance, because it is assumed that with the same genes and the same shared environment, the measure of the trait should be the same for each of the twin pair. So, if you take a group of twins – the larger the better – some will be very concordant and others less so. This means that there is variance in the measure of the trait in the sample, for example, on a test of numerical abilities. By comparing the variance in the concordance

---

of monozygotic (MZ) twins and dizygotic (DZ) twins, we can get an estimate of heritability. If the concordance is the same between the two groups, then there is little or no contribution of heritability, and the effects of the environment are key; if monozygotic twins are sufficiently more concordant than dizygotes, then there is a significant contribution of genetic factors. Using statistical methods of comparing the variances in the concordances between the two groups of twins, we can estimate the contributions of genetic factors, common and unique environmental factors.

This means that an index of heritability – usually written h^2 – is not an estimate of how much of an individual's phenotype is due to heredity, but rather an estimate of the proportion of variance in the sample of twins that can be attributed to genetic factors. It also does not tell you which genes are involved.

In some of the studies mentioned, a subsample of probands is selected, for example, children who are particularly bad at maths. For this approach, a different statistical method is employed, called DeFries–Fulker Extremes Analysis. This method also looks at the differences between MZ and DZ twins. In the sample, it would be expected that the proband's cotwin will be more like the mean of the whole sample – "regression towards the mean". If both MZ and DZ cotwins regress by the same amount, then it is inferred that the cause of maths disability is environmental since both twins are assumed to have the same environment; but, if the DZ cotwins regress more than MZ cotwins, this is evidence for a genetic effect.

The first study to use twins to estimate the heritability ("h^2") was carried out by a team at the Colorado Learning Disabilities Research Center led by John de Fries and Bruce Pennington, pioneers in this kind of work. They selected *monozygotic* (MZ) and *dizygotic* (DZ) twin pairs where one twin (the "proband") had a school history of maths problems and had a standardized maths score than was 1.5 standard deviations below the control sample (approximately the bottom 6%), and who had no other serious neurological, behavioural, or emotional problems, and whose IQ was at least 90 (that is, in the normal or superior range). They found a significant effect of heritability: MZ twin pairs were more concordant than DZ twin pairs, that is, it was more likely that both MZ twins had a maths learning disability, than with DZ twins. The estimate of heritability was .38. To be completely heritable the estimate would be 1, so most of the variance is attributable to common and unique environmental factors, such as home environment (see Chapter 8 for the effects of environmental factors on arithmetical competencies). One other interesting finding from this study, was that the heritability for maths was higher in twins who had both a maths disability and a reading disability (Alarcon et al., 1997). I deal with this issue of "co-morbidity" in more detail in Chapter 9 on assessment.

A more recent study took a different approach. Instead of identifying probands with dyscalculia or mathematical learning disability, they tested a large sample of 1,500 pairs of MZ and 1375 pairs of DZ seven-year-old same-sex twins using participants from the Twins Early Development Study, a large UK database of twins. Mathematical ability was assessed by teachers based on UK National Curriculum Key Stage 1 criteria for mathematical attainment. Reading and general cognitive abilities were tested using standardized test batteries. They found that about 30% of the genetic variance was specific to mathematics.

A second investigation by Yulia Kovas and her team at Goldsmith's College, University of London, used a web-based battery of tests of maths and reading on 2,596 pairs of ten-year-old twins from the Twins Early Development Study. Here, as with Alarcon et al. (1997), they selected a subsample of children who were particularly bad at maths (the lowest 15%). This required a different method of statistical analysis (DeFries–Fulker Extremes Analysis, see Box 7.1) (Kovas et al., 2007). They concluded that

> Both reading and mathematics disability are moderately heritable (47% and 43%, respectively) and show only modest shared environmental influence (16% and 20%) … [but there was a] genetic correlation of.67 between reading disability and mathematics disability, suggesting that they are affected largely by the same genetic factors.
>
> (p. 914)

The investigation used standardized maths and reading tests in which performance seemed heavily dependent on education – both formal and informal – so it is perhaps not surprising that factors that affected learning to read also affected learning arithmetic. There was no test of core competence such as a test of number sense.

However, the team carried out a more recent study specifically of the heritability of number sense. They tested 4,518 twins (2259 pairs): 836 monozygotic (MZ), 733 dizygotic same-sex (DZ), and 689 dizygotic opposite-sex (DZ) pairs, with a mean age of 16.6 years, drawn from Twins Early Development Study (Tosto et al., 2014). The number sense test they used was the same as the one in Figure 2.3a in Chapter 2, where the task is to say whether there are more blue or more yellow dots. You will remember the "distance effect"; that is, the bigger the proportional difference – "distance" – between the number of blue and yellow dots, the easier it is to get it right. There are individual differences, as we saw in Chapter 2: some people are good at this – for example, they can reliably discriminate a 20% difference, while others need a 40% difference to reliably get it right. The proportional difference is called the "Weber Fraction" after the German scientist who discovered the effect.

They found only modest heritability for number sense, with the biggest factor being non-shared environment (see Figure 7.1).

When the 4,000 twin pairs from the Twins Early Development Study reached the age of 12, a further investigation was carried out, again looking at the lowest

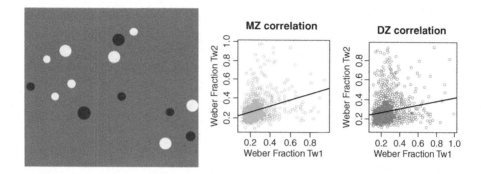

Figure 7.1 Testing number sense in twins. The stimuli are in the left panel, and the task is to say whether there are more blue or more yellow dots. The middle panel shows the correlation between the Weber Fraction (the ability) of each pair of MZ twins and the right panel shows the correlation between each pair of DZ twins. The correlations are modest, but MZ twins are more similar to each other than DZ twins suggesting heritability of number sense. From Tosto et al., 2014.

15% in reading and maths, along with tests of language and general cognitive ability (IQ). Again, there was a significant genetic influence on maths ability, as well as on reading, language and IQ (Haworth et al., 2009).

However, the authors of these studies stress that there is a very high correlation among all these measures, and have suggested that underlying this correlation are "generalist genes" that affect all aspects of cognitive ability, and disability. They add that non-shared environmental influences "operate as specialists", and contribute to being bad at maths, for example, but not at reading. Shared environment, by contrast, affects all the measures.

Because they have tested largely the same population of twins at eight, ten and 12 years, they are able to infer that "Continuity is genetic and change is environmental: Longitudinal analyses suggest that age-to-age stability is primarily mediated genetically, whereas the environment contributes to change from age to age" (Kovas et al., 2007, p. 1). Bear in mind that the sample of low attainment is the bottom 15%, while the best estimates of the prevalence of dyscalculia is 3.5–5% (see Chapter 3). This means that the sample will include learners who are bad at maths for many different reasons, and not just dyscalculia. The evidence presented in Figure 7.1 suggests that *number sense* is modestly heritable, but, as I discussed in Chapter 3, the test used here may not be the best way to identify the core ability that underlies arithmetic learning.

Overall, we can conclude from studies of twins that:

- For school performance on standardized tests of maths, there is *a significant specific genetic effect*, but there are also general genetic effects that the shape of school performance on measures of language and reading as well, and is linked to general cognitive ability.

- School performance on all the measures is affected by shared environment (see Chapter 5 for the effects of domain-general cognitive abilities and Chapter 8 for home and school factors).
- School performance on maths, but not reading, is affected by non-shared environment.

Gender

The most obvious genetic difference between individuals is gender, which determined by the sex chromosomes. Humans have one pair of sex chromosomes – in females the pair is designated by XX, where X indicates the female chromosome. One X is inherited from the mother and one from the father. In males, the pair is designated by XY, where they Y is inherited from the father. Humans also have 22 pairs of *autosomes*, which control the inheritance of all the characteristics except the sex-linked ones.

We can now ask the following questions about *sex-linkage* in maths ability:

- Are males better or worse at maths than females?
- Are there more males than females with the maths highest ability?
- Are there more males than females with dyscalculia?

Are males better than females?

It is certainly true that in the UK before the Second World War, boys used to be much better than girls at maths. This became a cause of concern resulting in several reports including a Royal Commission. There were many reasons for this, but perhaps the most important was that girls were taught in girls' schools by female teachers, few of whom had been to university and even fewer had done university-level maths. When I went to school in the 1950s and 1960s, secondary schools, especially "grammar" or high schools were typically single-sex. With the introduction by the Labour government of mixed comprehensive schools, all children were taught by the same teachers, and girls eventually did as well in maths exams as boys, as a recent review of school exams explains:

> There is little evidence of a male advantage in high school mathematics tests in either the US or the UK. In the US, "trivial differences" between boys' and girls' mathematics results have been found in all school years between Grade 2 (7–8 year olds) and Grade 11 (16–17 year olds).... At the end of high school, it is girls who have been achieving, on average, higher Grade Point Average points (in mathematics and science combined) than boys since at least the 1990s.... Similarly, the UK Department for Education and Skills' (2006) report on gender and education emphasises a *female advantage* amongst students gaining an A★–C grade in GSCE mathematics in England, although this pattern has changed from the pre-1991 pattern when males outperformed girls in the U.S.
>
> (Bramley et al., 2015, p. 3)

It is nevertheless worth noting, that in almost all other subjects, girls now significantly outperform boys in these exams.

Another way of exploring whether there is a sex-linked effect, is to compare mathematical abilities in different countries and different educational systems, so one can evaluate whether any gender difference is due to culture and other environmental factors – such as teachers and parents thinking that maths is more important for boys than for girls.

There are two such large international surveys where the same tests are given to boys and girls in each country. The better known are the studies carried out by a department of the Organisation of Economic Cooperation and Development, and known as the PISA studies (not after the Italian city, but an acronym for the Programme for International Student Assessment). Their most recent survey is summarized thus:

> Girls underperform in mathematics, compared with boys, in 38 of the 65 countries and economies that participated in PISA 2012; in OECD countries, girls underperform boys by an average of 11 points. However, this gender gap between the average 15-year-old boy and girl masks even wider gaps among the least and most able students. In most countries, the most able girls lag behind the most able boys in mathematics performance.
>
> (www.oecd.org/pisa/keyfindings/pisa-2012-results-overview.pdf)

Notice that boys are better in some countries but not in others. In fact, girls outperform boys significantly in five countries.

The second international study is called TIMSS – Trends in International Mathematics and Science Study. Like PISA, TIMSS took a representative sample of children – more than 600,000 in 63 countries – but unlike PISA, it took two age groups, fourth and eighth grade instead of 15-year-olds.

It summarises the gender effect, or lack of it, thus:

> Averaging mathematics achievement across countries, it is clear that there was little achievement difference between girls and boys (International Average: 490 vs. 491). Of the 50 countries at the fourth grade, 26 had no significant gender difference in mathematics achievement. Of the 24 remaining countries, 20 had small differences favoring boys, and four had relatively larger differences favoring girls (Qatar, Thailand, Oman, and Kuwait).

Another way of thinking about gender effects is to ask whether changes – including improvements – in the educational system affects boys and girls equally. TIMSS shows that it does. See Figure 7.2.

To summarise, there is basically no difference between males and females on average, when they are exposed to comparable teaching.

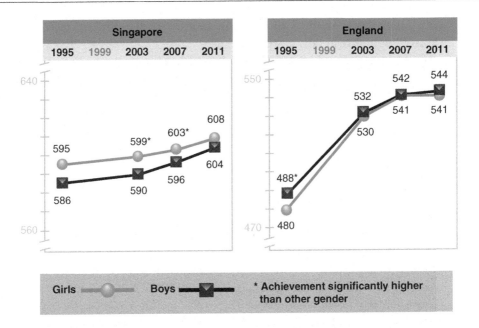

Figure 7.2 Changes in average performance in school children two countries tested by TIMSS. On the whole, the improvements in each country are equivalent for boys and girls. Notice that girls in Singapore were significantly better than boys in 2003 and 2007.

From Mullis et al., 2012.

Are there more males than females with the maths highest ability?

The PISA study finds the following:

> Gender gaps in drive, motivation and self-beliefs are particularly worrying because these factors are essential if students are to achieve at the highest levels; and the relationship between drive, motivation and mathematics-related self-beliefs on the one hand, and mathematics performance on the other, is particularly strong at the top of the performance distribution. Unless girls believe that they can achieve at the highest levels, they will not be able to do so.

In fact, many studies have found a disproportionate number of males at the top end of the ability range.

> Despite a female advantage in school results, males in the U.S show a persistent trend to perform better in high-stakes examinations such as in the mathematics sections of the SAT and ACT examinations which are taken for entry to universities in the U.S.

> (Bramley et al., 2015)

Another line of research has attempted to assess whether sex-linked characteristics contribute to this high-level performance. U.S. psychologist Caroline Benbow and her colleagues have found a significant advantage for talented 12–13 year old boys over girls at the upper end of the ability range, as measured by SAT-M (Scholastic Aptitude Test – Mathematics), while SAT-V (Verbal) showed no comparable difference (see Benbow, 1988, for a review). Benbow argues that the sex difference cannot be explained in terms of "environmental" hypotheses to do with attitudes, confidence, or teaching. She argues rather that a combination of biological differences between the sexes is the cause, in particular a more bilateral neural representation of cognitive functions in the female brain (see below).

However, there have been very few studies of the brain systems of expert calculators. Benbow, O'Boyle and colleagues (e.g. Alexander et al., 1996; O'Boyle et al., 1995; O'Boyle et al., 1994; Singh & O'Boyle, 2004) have investigated mathematically gifted children and adolescents, with special reference to gender and brain organisation. In general, they have found more right-hemisphere involvement in a range of tasks, though, curiously, mathematical tasks themselves have not been studied.

The differences between boys and girls in SAT-M performance appears to follow from the larger variance in boys' scores, which would allow reliable differences at the top end of the range even if the mean score for girls were the same or even higher than for boys. However, the greater variance in males seems not to be universal. In some populations, there are more girls at the highest levels of school maths attainment than boys, and, in many, including TIMSS, there is no significant difference in the variances. In any case, the finding of a larger variance in male performance, on a whole range of abilities, not just maths, with more boys at the bottom as well as the top ends of the range, still needs an explanation.

Nevertheless, when one looks at the means, girls in England easily outperform boys in all subjects at all ages. There is one exception to this general rule: mathematics. Girls are only just outperforming boys, as noted above.

Are there more males than females with dyscalculia?
In our study of 11,500 children in Havana, dyscalculia was defined as having very poor arithmetic for their age *plus* a core deficit in number sense (see Chapter 4). There was no gender effect for those children who just had poor arithmetic alone, but there was a big and significant gender effect for dyscalculia: 2.4 males to 1 female fell into this category.

Genetic anomalies

For another way of looking for the effects of genetics, I start with considering conditions that show the core deficit. Arithmetical impairments and *core deficits* have been observed in many genetic conditions:

- Turner's syndrome (TS) (Braundet et al., 2004)
- Cerebral palsy (CP) (Arp & Fagard, 2005; Arp et al., 2006)

- Velocardiofacial syndrome (VCFS – also known as Chromosome 22q11.2 Deletion syndrome, or DS22q11.2) (De Smedt et al., 2007)
- Fragile X syndrome (FXS) (Mazzocco & McCloskey, 2005)
- Williams syndrome (WS) (Paterson et al., 2006)

I want to start with one condition that is not – indeed cannot be inherited – namely Turner's Syndrome (TS). This condition affects 1 in 2,000 live births. It affects only females since it is a sporadic partial or total absence of one of the two X chromosomes, so as a result they are infertile. The most extensive studies have involved the 45X karyotype – that is, females lacking one X chromosome. Unlike the other conditions in the list, TS females are typically cognitively in the normal range except for arithmetic.

For example, one study of adult 45X TS, found them to be normal on counting, and as *accurate* as matched controls on dot enumeration, simple addition, subtraction and division; however, they were significantly *slower* on all the tasks (Bruandet et al., 2004).

Similarly, in our study of seven 45X TS females from 17 to 27 years, we also found them to be slower on addition, subtraction, and multiplication. They were also much slower on a test of core number sense – dot enumeration. But they were not just slow at everything: they were entirely normal on a simple reaction time test. That is, they were slower only when it came to numbers, even though three out of the seven managed to pass formal maths exams. In fact, three of the seven participants in our study achieved an A at GCSE (16 years) and, one, a science teacher passed Advanced Level mathematics at school (Butterworth et al., 1999).

Preterm and very low birthweight

Children born very preterm (VP, <32weeks gestational age) or extremely preterm (EP, <26 weeks) or with very low birth-weight (VLBW, <1500g) are likely to do badly at school, and especially at maths (Isaacs et al., 2001) and see (Simms et al., 2013a) for a review. This is the case when tested at a wide range of ages and on a wide range of standardized maths tests, and at a variety of VP, EP and VLBW. Although these children often have poor domain-general cognitive capacities as measured by IQ tests, the difficulties in maths are not accounted for by lower IQ (Simms et al., 2013a).

There appears to be a domain-specific deficit. A team at Leicester University has used a numerosity comparison task similar to those in Figure 2.1 and a number line task similar to that in Figure 2.6. They found that these children are poorer on these tasks, and that performance on these tasks predicted performance on standardized maths tasks. However, individual differences in domain-general skills were also important, in fact more so in the typical population. Simms et al. (2013a) conclude that "the mathematics difficulties associated with preterm birth are likely to be the result of a complex interplay between both domain-specific and domain-general factors." (Simms et al., 2013b) p460.

A team at the UCL Institute of Child Health led by Elizabeth Isaacs and Alan Lucas have shown VLBW is associated with reduced grey matter in the region of the parietal lobe (Isaacs et al., 2001) that we now know supports basic numerical processing (Castelli et al., 2006) (see Chapter 6).

However, the reasons and consequences of VLBW are complex, since there are often medical complications, such as respiratory disease and hypoglycaemia, and nutritional variables, both intrauterine and in the first few months, may play a role (Isaacs et al., 2001).

Foetal alcohol syndrome (FAS)

A diagnosis of FAS is normally based on three criteria:

> (1) a growth deficiency of prenatal origin for height or weight; (2) a pattern of specific minor anomalies that includes characteristic facial features and (3) central nervous system dysfunction, including microcephaly, delayed development, hyperactivity, attention deficits, learning disabilities, intellectual deficits, and so forth.… Patients are often described as having possible Fetal Alcohol Effects (FAE) when they are heavily exposed to alcohol *in utero* and have some, but not all, of the hallmark features of FAS.
>
> (Kopera-Frye et al., 1996)

A UK government review notes that "Avoidance of alcohol exposure during pre-natal development is particularly important since "foetal alcohol syndrome" is currently recognised as the most common known environmental cause of mental retardation, affecting from 1 to 7 per 1000 live-born infants" (Kirkwood et al., 2010).

The review also points out that "[a] continuing controversy involves the degree to which the deficits derive from prenatal alcohol exposure, rather than from neglectful and/or nonstimulating environments often provided by alcoholic mothers who continue to drink". The effects of maternal alcohol consumption can vary widely, depending on when in the gestation period and how much alcohol is consumed and hence FAS is sometimes called "Foetal alcohol spectrum disorders" – FASD (e.g. Mattson et al., 2011).

Among the cognitive consequences of maternal alcohol consumption are lower general intelligence, poorer executive function and problem-solving, weaker response inhibition, reduced working memory and long-term memory, language difficulties, poorer visuo-spatial ability, motor skills, and attention (Mattson et al., 2011). Identifying specific, and especially core deficits, in mathematics is therefore a challenge. However, one recent review puts it like this: "Mathematics has emerged as a specific area of weakness.… Alcohol-exposed children consistently perform lower than controls on measures of global mathematics achievement" (Mattson et al., 2011).

A study by Dehaene and colleagues showed in 29 patients with FAS, or with Foetal Alcohol Effects, a clear deficit in calculation and estimation, while other number tasks such as reading numbers or selecting the larger of two digits were within the normal range. Now calculation requires the involvement of the frontal lobes as well as the parietal lobes, as we saw in Chapter 6. The estimation test was based on a test specifically designed to assess frontal lobe function (Shallice & Evans, 1978). Here the exact answer is unlikely to be known, and is not required; rather it should be in the "acceptable range". This demands reasoning from different bits of evidence: What is the length of an average man's spine? (acceptable range 2–4 feet; patient range: 1–24 feet) How long does it take to cook a fish? (7–30 minutes; 2.5 minutes–5 hours); How fast do racehorses gallop? (10–50 mph; 3–2,000 mph). These FAS patients did not therefore seem to have core deficit, but rather poor arithmetical competence as a result of domain-general cognitive difficulties.

What about the brains of FAS sufferers? "Recent neuroimaging studies support neuropsychological findings and have shown that children with FASD show abnormalities in regions thought to be important in mathematical processing, such as left and right parietal regions and the medial frontal gyrus" (Mattson et al., 2011).

It turns out that both grey matter and white matter volumes are closely related to cognitive function in FASD, while this isn't the case in typical development (Gautam et al., 2014).

Overall, the effects of FAS seems to give rise to the type of low numeracy and low mathematical attainment that was described in Chapter 5 rather than true dyscalculia, that is, the type caused by the core deficit described in Chapter 4.

Gerstmann's Syndrome: the role of fingers

The close association between fingers and arithmetic in early years has been well established. For example, researchers have reported that preschool children (Fuson, 1988; Gelman & Gallistel, 2004), and children in the first years of school use their fingers to support calculation (Reeve et al., in prep). Geary, Hoard, Byrd-Craven, and Catherine DeSoto (2004) found that American kindergarteners used fingers on 29% of addition trials where the sum was <11, and 76% of trials where it was >10. In first and second grade, they were still using fingers on 35% of trials. This pattern is not universal: Chinese children of the same age did not use fingers at all (Geary et al., 1996). Geary et al. note that "[t]he use of fingers during counting appears to be a working memory aid that allows the child to keep track of the addends physically, rather than mentally, during the process of counting".

Finger agnosia is where a child has difficulty mentally representing his or her fingers. So that they have difficulty accurately reporting which finger has been touched without seeing (see Figure 7.3). This has been associated with poor early arithmetic (Fayol et al., 1998; Reeve & Humberstone, 2011). What is

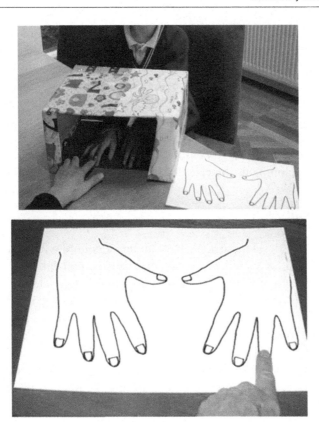

Figure 7.3 A method used for testing for finger agnosia. The child is touched on one finger and is required to point to the finger touched on the diagram of the hands (Reeve & Humberstone, 2011). Other methods require the child to report the finger touched, for example, to say "right index" (Kinsbourne & Warrington, 1963).

more, training children to represent their fingers more accurately, helps the development of arithmetic, so there does appear to be a causal relationship of some sort between finger representation and arithmetical development (Bafalluy & Noël, 2008).

Josef Gerstmann, an Austrian neurologist, was well aware of the relationships between numbers, space and the body, and he observed in his patients that disorders of one often co-occurred with disorders of the others. The Gerstmann syndrome, as it is now known, is a combination of four impairments, two involving symbol systems (dyscalculia and dysgraphia) and two involving the representation of the body (left-right disorientation and finger agnosia). Gerstmann himself thought that the key to the syndrome was an impaired "body schema", that showed up in the left-right disorientation, and particularly in finger agnosia because this required a very detailed representation. He associated this syndrome with damage to the *left parietal lobe*, and subsequent research has confirmed this (Rusconi et al., 2009; Rusconi et al., 2005).

In the early 1960s, scientists at the National Hospital for Neurology in London were the first to report developmental cases who had all four symptoms but no detectable neurological damage (Kinsbourne & Warrington, 1963). Subsequent research has found cases with neural abnormality and co-occurring cognitive symptoms, but many, perhaps most, cases showed no neurological signs and no cognitive impairments. There also seems to be no causal genetic factor.

So although Gerstmann's proposal has led to a greater interest in the relationship between the body – "embodied cognition" – especially fingers and arithmetical development, the cause of the syndrome is still enigmatic.

Acquired acalculia

The typically developing adult in a numerate culture will acquire a wide range of mathematical competences that depend in large part on educational opportunity. We know that competent adults, even very competent adults, depend on the same fronto-parietal network as the less able. There is some evidence that professional mathematicians show greater grey matter density in the left parietal lobe than non-mathematicians and that the increase in density is proportional to the number of years that they have been practicing as university-level mathematicians (Aydin et al., 2007). There is also evidence that exceptional calculators recruit additional neural resources to support greater working memory load imposed by complex calculations (Pesenti, 2005; Pesenti et al., 1999; Pesenti et al., 2001). Of course, good mathematicians and expert calculators know far more mathematics than the rest of us, and this has to be stored somewhere in the brain.

Now acquired acalculia is called "acquired" because a normally developed network has *acquired* damage from traumatic brain injury, cardio-vascular disease affecting the brain (stroke), brain tumour, and a range of diseases affecting the brain, such as the dementias. A note on terminology: "Acalculia" is the term most often used in adult neuropsychology and "dyscalculia" in the developmental literature.

Acquired acalculia is like developmental dyscalculia in two ways:

- It can be completely selective. That is, the patient's other cognitive functions may be entirely normal and indeed intact. For example, severe acalculia can be found in patients who have normal reasoning, intelligence, memory, and symbolic abilities, and yet be unable to deal with numbers above four, and indeed deal with numbers four and below abnormally (Cipolotti et al., 1991). We can also find patients with the opposite pattern – preserved calculation, but severe impairments in memory and language (Cappelletti et al., 2001).
- On the other hand, it can go along with other cognitive impairments, especially in cases of degenerative diseases (Cappelletti et al., 2012; Semenza et al., 2014), just as dyscalculia can co-occur with other cognitive difficulties.

However, there is one important difference. In dyscalculia, the core deficit in the number module is easily identified using a test for number sense, such as dot enumeration or numerosity comparison (see Chapter 4). This deficit prevents the numerical system from developing normally. In acquired acalculia, the numerical system has usually developed normally, that is without the core deficit, and is complex. In a review of the literature, my colleague Marinella Cappelletti, a neuropsychologist at Goldsmith's College University of London, summarises the basic components of the "normal" number system as follows:

- *The number semantic system* that includes symbolic quantity – counting words and digits, non-symbolic quantity – the numerosity of sets of objects, arithmetical conceptual knowledge – the laws of arithmetic, for example, and number encyclopaedic knowledge – Levis 501, 2001 Space Odyssey, historical dates, TV channels, phone numbers and so on.
- *Processes* such as counting, reading numbers, writing numbers, retrieving arithmetical facts, calculating.

What Cappelletti shows in this review is that each of these components can be selectively affected by brain damage. Someone may be able to retrieve, say, multiplication facts, but not understand that a x b is the same as b x a (see patient JG below); they may be able to multiply but not add, or add but not multiply, read numbers but not be able to write them, or write them but not be able read to read them; to calculate with digits that have been read and write the solution but not be able read digits aloud, or write digits to dictation (Cipolotti & Butterworth, 1995). For systematic reviews of these phenomena see Cappelletti (2015) and (Cipolotti & van Harskamp, 2001).

What these dissociations demonstrate is that, in a numerate society, the adult number system is "modular", that is, it consists of relatively independent components, each of which can be preserved or impaired selectively. This is supported by neuroimaging studies that show somewhat different patterns of activation for each of the four arithmetical operations (Arsalidou & Taylor, 2011), and see Chapter 6.

This means that assessment of these patients will be very different from that of developmental dyscalculic learners. Each type of knowledge and each type of process will need to be assessed separately. Fortunately, there is a handy protocol for making the initial assessment called Numerical Activities of Daily Living (Semenza et al., 2014).

In Chapter 6, we saw that dyscalculia was associated with specific abnormalities in the brain, in particular, in reduced grey matter in the left intraparietal sulcus, and possibly in the white matter connections to and from this region which have arisen as the result of a developmental process, perhaps due to genetic causes, perhaps from some other cause. The question therefore arises as to whether brain damage later in life can affect the brain in such a way as to mimic this abnormal neural development.

There are some candidates. For example, patient JG suffered a left parietal tumour and her symptoms were reported by my colleague Margarete Delazer and the neurologist Thomas Benke at the University Neurology Clinic in Innsbruck in a paper with the title *Arithmetic facts without meaning* (Delazer & Benke, 1997). The title really tells it all. The tumour – a glioblastoma - gave rise to Gerstmann's Syndrome which comprises four deficits: agraphia (an inability to write), left–right orientation, finger agnosia (a defective mental representation of her fingers such that she could not tell which of her fingers was being touched unless she was allowed to see), and acalculia. For single digit multiplication she scored 59 out of 64, but for single digit addition, only 28 out of 64, subtraction, 12 out of 38, division, zero. On a standard multidigit addition and subtraction test, she scored zero. She was completely unable to use paper and pencil, number lines or fingers to work out multiplication problems, even those she could retrieve from memory. She was also completely unable to solve problems using arithmetical principles (see Table 7.1).

So, although JG could remember multiplication facts – perhaps stored in memory as strings of words (remember how these facts are learned in school) – she

Table 7.1 Patient JG's attempts to use arithmetical principles to solve problems. For example, she was presented with 13 + 9 = 22 and asked to solve 9 + 13.

Arithmetic Principles Task

	J.G. n correct	Controls % correct	Given problem	Unknown problem
Addition				
Commutativity	1/3	93.3%	13 + 9 = 22	9 + 13 ?
a + 1 principle	0/3	100%	13 + 9 = 22	14 + 9?
a − 1 principle	0/3	100%	13 + 9 = 22	12 + 9?
10a + 10b principle	0/3	93.3%	13 + 9 = 22	130 + 90 ?
Addition/subtraction inverse principle	0/3	86.7%	13 + 9 = 22	22 − 9 ?
Multiplication				
Commutativity	0/3	100%	12 × 4 = 48	4 × 12 ?
Repeated add.	0/3	100%	2 × 4 = 48	12 + 12 + 12 + 12?
10a × 10b principle	0/3	46.7%	2 × 4 = 48	120 × 40 ?
a − 1 principle	0/3	93.3%	2 × 4 = 48	11 × 4 ?
Multiplication/division inverse principle	0/3	100%	2 × 4 = 48	48 : 4 ?

Note - Unknown problems should be derived from given ones, the table gives examples for each condition. Controls had to answer more difficult problems (based on the same principles), since they could answer small problems by calculating the result.

didn't seem to be able to understand what the numbers meant and how numbers are relatable by arithmetical principles. One other test reinforces this conclusion: she was asked to compose numbers from poker chips with values 1, 2, 5, 10, 20, 50, 100. Here are some examples of her answers: target 12, solution 5 5 5 2 2 2 2 2 2; target 38, solution 10 10 10 5 1 1.

Did she therefore have a core deficit? This isn't completely clear. She could do dot enumeration fairly accurately, but was much slower than controls. However, she was able select the larger of two digits accurately with a normal distance effect.

A more extreme case was reported by Lisa Cipolotti, neurologist Gianfranco Denes and me. Patient CG suffered a cerebral vascular accident (stroke) that caused a lesion in the left fronto-parietal region – the number network (Cipolotti et al., 1991). Despite normal IQ, she was unable to carry out the simplest calculation if it contained a number above four. She was unable to subitize, and counted aloud the dots from one to four. Numerosity comparison was impossible for numerosities greater than four, as was comparison of digits. Similarly, she was unable to put cards with numbers of dots into an ascending sequence. It turned out that she also had trouble with other sequences, such as days of the week, months of the year or the alphabet.

She was quite unable to recall number facts, not only from arithmetic, but the number of days in the week or in a year, or her age, her shoe size, or her address.

This does, in one way, look like dyscalculia. It is an isolated disability: she had good knowledge of non-numerical symbols, her reasoning was competent, and her IQ was average. Although she could not compare numbers or the numerosities of two arrays of objects, she was able to compare the physical sizes of objects when presented as pictures: that is, she could say that an elephant was bigger than a mouse even when their pictures were the same size. A stronger test, though, would have been to see if she could relearn the meanings of numbers, and the arithmetical facts and principles which depend on them. To the extent that they are based on the core capacity, on the number module, in the parietal lobe, this should be very difficult. Unfortunately, we did not have the opportunity to test this.

Summary

- Twin studies show that there is a substantial heritable component in dyscalculia, though good candidate genes are still to be discovered
- Not all cases of dyscalculia will be inherited, though the proportion is not yet known; some are due to genetic mutations, including those, like Turner's Syndrome, that cannot be inherited. Individuals suffering these conditions typically have a core deficit.
- Disturbances to pregnancy including pre-term birth and foetal alcohol syndrome can also lead to dyscalculia.
- Brain damage in adulthood can lead to severe impairments in arithmetical competence, but with patterns of deficit different from dyscalculia.

References

Alarcon, M., Defries, J., Gillis Light, J., & Pennington, B. (1997). A twin study of mathematics disability. *Journal of Learning Disabilities*, 30, 617–623.

Alexander, J. E., O'Boyle, M. W., & Benbow, C. P. (1996). Developmentally advanced EEG alpha power in gifted male and female adolescents. *International Journal of Psychophysiology*, 23, 25–31.

Arp, S., & Fagard, J. (2005). What impairs subitizing in cerebral palsied children? *Developmental Psychobiology*, 47(1), 89–102.

Arp, S., Taranne, P., & Fagard, J. (2006). Global perception of small numerosities (subitizing) in cerebral-palsied children. *Journal of Clinical and Experimental Neuropsychology*, 28, 405–419.

Arsalidou, M., & Taylor, M. J. (2011). Is 2+2=4? Meta-analyses of brain areas needed for numbers and calculations. *NeuroImage*, 54(3), 2382–2393. doi: 10.1016/j.neuroimage. 2010.10.009

Aydin, K., Ucar, A., Oguz, K. K., Okur, O. O., Agayev, A., Unal, Z., Yilmaz, S., & Ozturk, S. (2007). Increased gray matter density in the parietal cortex of mathematicians: A Voxel-Based Morphometry study. *American Journal of Neuroradiology*, 28, 1859–1864.

Bafalluy, M. G., & Noël, M.-P. (2008). Does finger training increase young children's numerical performance? *Cortex*, 44, 368–375. doi: 10.1016/j.cortex.2007.08.020

Benbow, C. P. (1988). Sex differences in mathematical reasoning ability in intellectually talented preadolescents: Their nature, effects, and possible causes. *Behavioral and Brain Sciences*, 11(2), 169–183.

Bramley, T., Vidal Rodeiro, C. L., & Vitello, S. (2015). *Gender differences in GCSE:* Cambridge Assessment Research Report. Cambridge, UK: Cambridge Assessment.

Braundet, M., Molko, N., Cohen, L., & Dehaene, S. (2004). A cognitive characterization of dyscalculia in Turner syndrome. *Neuropsychologia*, 42, 288–298.

Butterworth, B., Granà, A., Piazza, M., Girelli, L., Price, C., & Skuse, D. (1999). Language and the origins of number skills: karyotypic differences in Turner's syndrome. *Brain & Language*, 69, 486–488.

Cappelletti, M., Butterworth, B., & Kopelman, M. (2001). Spared numerical abilities in a case of semantic dementia. *Neuropsychologia*, 39, 1224–1239.

Cappelletti, M., Butterworth, B., & Kopelman, M. (2012). Numeracy Skills in Patients With Degenerative Disorders and Focal Brain Lesions: A Neuropsychological Investigation. *Neuropsychology*, 26(1), 1–19. doi: 10.1037/a0026328

Castelli, F., Glaser, D. E., & Butterworth, B. (2006). Discrete and analogue quantity processing in the parietal lobe: A functional MRI study. *Proceedings of the National Academy of Sciences of the United States of America*, 103(12), 4693–4698.

Cipolotti, L., & Butterworth, B. (1995). Toward a multiroute model of number processing: Impaired number transcoding with preserved calculation skills. *Journal of Experimental Psychology: General*, 124, 375–390.

Cipolotti, L., & van Harskamp, N. (2001). Disturbances of number processing and calculation. In R. S. Berndt (Ed.), *Handbook of Neuropsychology* (2nd. ed., Vol. 3, pp. 305–334). Amsterdam: Elsevier Science.

Cipolotti, L., Butterworth, B., & Denes, G. (1991). A specific deficit for numbers in a case of dense acalculia. *Brain*, 114, 2619–2637.

De Smedt, B., Swillen, A., Devriendt, K., Fryns, J. P., Verschaffel, L., & Ghesquiere, P. (2007). Mathematical disabilities in children with velo-cardio-facial syndrome. *Neuropsychologia*, 45(5), 885–895.

Delazer, M., & Benke, T. (1997). Arithmetic facts without meaning. *Cortex*, 33, 697–710.

Fayol, M., Barrouillet, P., & Marinthe, C. (1998). Predicting arithmetical achievement from neuro-psychological performance: A longitudinal study. *Cognition*, 68, 63–70.

Fuson, K. C. (1988). *Children's Counting and Concepts of Number*. New York: Springer Verlag.

Gautam, P., Nuñez, S. C., Narr, K. L., Kan, E. C., & Sowell, E. R. (2014). Effects of prenatal alcohol exposure on the development of white matter volume and change in executive function. *NeuroImage: Clinical*, 5, 19–27. doi: 10.1016/j.nicl.2014.05.010

Geary, D. C., Bow-Thomas, C. C., Liu, F., & Siegler, R. S. (1996). Development of Arithmetical Competencies in Chinese and American Children: Influence of Age, Language, and Schooling. *Child Development*, 67(5), 2022–2044.

Geary, D. C., Hoard, M. K., Byrd-Craven, J., & Catherine DeSoto, M. (2004). Strategy choices in simple and complex addition: Contributions of working memory and counting knowledge for children with mathematical disability. *Journal of Experimental Child Psychology*, 88(2), 121–151. doi: 10.1016/j.jecp.2004.03.002

Gelman, R., & Gallistel, C. R. (2004). Language and the origin of numerical concepts. *Science*, 306, 441–443.

Haworth, C. M. A., Kovas, Y., Harlaar, N., Hayiou-Thomas, M. E., Petrill, S. A., Dale, P. S., & Plomin, R. (2009). Generalist genes and learning disabilities: a multivariate genetic analysis of low performance in reading, mathematics, language and general cognitive ability in a sample of 8000 12-year-old twins. *Journal of Child Psychology and Psychiatry*, 50(10), 1318–1325. doi: 10.1111/j.1469–7610.2009.02114.x

Isaacs, E. B., Edmonds, C. J., Lucas, A., & Gadian, D. G. (2001). Calculation difficulties in children of very low birthweight: A neural correlate. *Brain*, 124, 1701–1707.

Kinsbourne, M., & Warrington, E. K. (1963). The developmental Gerstmann Syndrome. *Annals of Neurology*, 8, 490–501.

Kirkwood, T., Bond, J., May, C., McKeith, I., & Teh, M.-M. (2010). Mental capital and well-being through life: Future challenges. *Mental Capital and Well-Being*, 3–53.

Kopera-Frye, K., Dehaene, S., & Streissguth, A. P. (1996). Impairments of number processing induced by prenatal alcohol exposure. *Neuropsychologia*, 34(12), 1187–1196. doi: http://dx.doi.org/10.1016/0028-3932(96)00043-7

Kovas, Y., Haworth, C. M., Dale, P. S., & Plomin, R. (2007). The genetic and environmental origins of learning abilities and disabilities in the early school years. *Monograph of the Society for Research in Child Development*, 72(3), 1–144.

Kovas, Y., Haworth, C. M. A., Harlaar, N., Petrill, S. A., & Plomin, R. (2007). Overlap and specificity of genetic and environmental influences on reading and mathematics disability in 10 year-old twins. *Journal of Child Psychology and Psychiatry*, 48(9), 914–922.

Mattson, S. N., Crocker, N., & Nguyen, T. T. (2011). Fetal Alcohol Spectrum Disorders: Neuropsychological and Behavioral Features. *Neuropsychology Review*, 21(2), 81–101. doi: 10.1007/s11065-011-9167–9

Mazzocco, M. M. M., & McCloskey, M. (2005). Math performance in girls with Turner or Fragile X syndrome. In J. I. D. Campbell (Ed.), *Handbook of Mathematical Cognition* (pp. 269–297). New York: Psychology Press.

Mullis, I. V. S., Martin, M. O., Foy, P., & Arora, A. (2012). *TIMSS 2011 International Results in Mathematics*. Chestnut Hill, MA, USA; Amsterdam, the Netherlands. TIMSS & PIRLS

International Study Center, Lynch School of Education, Boston College and International Association for the Evaluation of Educational Achievement (IEA) IEA Secretariat.

O'Boyle, M. W., Benbow, C. P., & Alexander, J. E. (1995). ex differences, hemispheric laterality, and associated brain activity in the intellectually gifted. *Developmental Neuropsychology*, 11(4), 415–443.

O'Boyle, M. W., Gill, H. S., Benbow, C. P., & Alexander, J. E. (1994). Concurrent finger-tapping in mathematically gifted males - evidence for enhanced right-hemisphere involvement during linguistic processing. *Cortex*, 30(3), 519–526.

Paterson, S. J., Girelli, L., Butterworth, B., & Karmiloff-Smith, A. (2006). Are numerical impairments syndrome specific? Evidence from Williams Syndrome and Down's Syndrome. *Journal of Child Psychology & Psychiatry*, 47(2), 190–204.

Pesenti, M. (2005). Calculation abilities in expert calculators. In J. I. D. Campbell (Ed.), *Handbook of Mathematical Cognition* (pp. 413–430). Hove: Psychology Press.

Pesenti, M., Seron, X., Samson, D., & Duroux, B. (1999). Basic and exceptional calculation abilities in a calculating prodigy: a case study. *Mathematical Cognition*, 5, 97–148.

Pesenti, M., Zago, L., Crivello, F., Mellet, E., Samson, D., Duroux, B., . . . Tzourio-Mazoyer, N. (2001). Mental calculation expertise in a prodigy is sustained by right prefrontal and medial-temporal areas. *Nature Neuroscience*, 4(1), 103–107.

Reeve, R., & Humberstone, J. (2011). Five- to 7-Year-Olds' Finger Gnosia and Calculation Abilities. *Frontiers in Psychology*, 2. doi: 10.3389/fpsyg.2011.00359

Reeve, R., Reynolds, F., Humberstone, J., & Butterworth, B. (in prep). Fingers and numbers: developmental pathways.

Rusconi, E., Walsh, V., & Butterworth, B. (2005). Dexterity with Numbers: rTMS Over Left Angular Gyrus Disrupts Finger Gnosis and Number Processing. *Neuropsychologia*, 43(11), 1609–1624.

Rusconi, E., Pinel, P., Eger, E., LeBihan, D., Thirion, B., Dehaene, S., & Kleinschmidt, A. (2009). A disconnection account of Gerstmann syndrome: Functional neuroanatomy evidence. *Annals of Neurology*, 66(5), 654–662. doi: 10.1002/ana.21776

Semenza, C., Meneghello, F., Arcara, G., Burgio, F., Gnoato, F., Facchini, S., Benavides-Varela, S., Clementi, M., & Butterworth, B. (2014). A new clinical tool for assessing numerical abilities in neurological diseases: Numerical Activities of Daily Living. *Frontiers in Aging Neuroscience*, 6. doi: 10.3389/fnagi.2014.00112

Shallice, T., & Evans, M. E. (1978). The involvement of the frontal lobes in cognitive estimation. *Cortex*, 14, 294–303.

Simms, V., Cragg, L., Gilmore, C., Marlow, N., & Johnson, S. (2013a). Mathematics difficulties in children born very preterm: current research and future directions. *Archives of Disease in Childhood – Fetal and Neonatal Edition*.

Simms, V., Gilmore, C., Cragg, L., Marlow, N., Wolke, D., & Johnson, S. (2013b). Mathematics difficulties in extremely preterm children: evidence of a specific deficit in basic mathematics processing. *Pediatr Res*, 73(2), 236–244.

Singh, H., & O'Boyle, M. W. (2004). Interhemispheric interaction during global-local processing in mathematically gifted adolescents, average-ability youth, and college students. *Neuropsychology*, 18(2), 371–377.

Tosto, M. G., Petrill, S. A., Halberda, J., Trzaskowski, M., Tikhomirova, T. N., Bogdanova, O. Y., Ly, R., Wilmer, J. B., Naiman, D. Q., Germine, L., Plomin, R., & Kovas, Y. (2014). Why do we differ in number sense? Evidence from a genetically sensitive investigation. *Intelligence*, 43, 35–46. doi: http://dx.doi.org/10.1016/j.intell.2013.12.007

CHAPTER

8

Society, school, and home

LEVEL OF EXPLANATION	MEASURES	EDUCATIONAL CONTEXT
BEHAVIOURAL	Number sense Chapter 2	**Society, school, and home**
COGNITIVE	Starter kit for learning arithmetic Chapter 3 Core deficit as the cause of dyscalculia Chapter 4	**Chapter 8** Assessment Chapter 9
	Development of arithmetic Chapter 5	Intervention Chapter 10
NEURAL	Brain structures and functions Chapter 6	Policy Chapter 11
	GENETIC AND OTHER CAUSES Chapter 7	

When children start school, they already show great individual differences in numerical competence. As well as domain-general cognitive factors (see Chapter 5) and domain-specific cognitive factors – core capacity or core deficit (see Chapters 3 and 4), there will be environmental factors such as social, economic, and parental education. "All these factors interact and it is difficult to determine their influence separately or together" (Benavides-Varela et al., 2016). These factors may also indirectly affect the quality of the formal educational environment since well-off parents can afford better schools for their children by buying private education or by buying a home in the catchment area of a better state school.

How children begin school is known to affect how they will continue.

> Children who start school with poor knowledge and skills in … numeracy … are unlikely to catch up to their peers. Individual differences in … numeracy skills are evident at school entry – prior to formal instruction—suggesting that children acquire fundamental skills at home.
>
> (Skwarchuk et al., 2014)

All this is well-known and has particular relevance to mathematical development (Melhuish et al., 2008). In this chapter, I want to focus on whether any environmental influences can give rise to dyscalculia rather than just poor progress and low numeracy. This is a very difficult issue. We know that dyscalculics have a core deficit in understanding basic numerical concepts (Chapter 4); we know that there is a heritable component (Chapter 7); we know that genetic anomalies, such as Turner's Syndrome, can give rise to it (Chapter 7); we know that it can persist into adulthood (Chapter 1); we know that dyscalculics have atypical brains (Chapter 6); we know that genes, perinatal problems (prematurity, foetal alcohol syndrome) affect brain development (Chapter 7); but we also know that the brain changes as we get older and it changes in response to experiences ("brain plasticity") (Shaw et al., 2006). This raises the interesting possibility that inappropriate numerical experiences, in particular lack of such experiences, can have similar effects on the brain as genetics and thereby result in dyscalculia. It also raises the possibility that appropriate experiences can ameliorate it (see Chapter 10 on intervention).

Society

There is now extensive evidence from two very large international surveys, PISA and TIMSS, about the effects of social factors on mathematical attainment (Mullis et al., 2012; OECD, 2016). Summarising a mass of data, the factors that both surveys identify, that inhibit arithmetical development both between and within nations, are poverty, poor nutrition, poor parental education, unhappiness at school and inequality.

Inequality is particularly interesting. For PISA, inequality is measured by the effect of socio-economic status (SES), where equitable societies, those with the smallest effect of SES, also tend to do best (OECD, 2016, p. 8; OECD, 2013, pp. 13, 28).

Looking more closely at the UK, a report from the Joseph Rowntree Foundation surveys the relationship between poverty and education. It notes that some 15% of children in England are classified as having Special Educational Needs and Disability (SEND), with 2.8% having a "statement" of special needs or an equivalent, that is official recognition and additional help. The Department for Education statistics show a clear link between SEND and children living in poverty. One way of identifying poverty is if the child is entitled to free school meals. In England, 29% of these children are identified as having SEND and this means that SEND children are twice as prevalent among disadvantaged pupils as among their less disadvantaged peers (Shaw et al., 2016). However, the report says nothing specifically about numeracy or dyscalculia.

Worldwide, and unsurprisingly, the children from the poorest families do significantly worse on cognitive tests, and have worse lifetime outcomes than their wealthier compatriots (Grantham-McGregor et al., 2007). Again, little attention has been paid specifically to numeracy difficulties. One study that looked at mathematics shows a clear relationship between PISA maths scores and poverty,

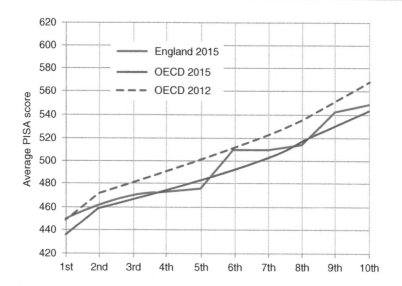

Figure 8.1 Parental income in deciles (tenths) from the poorest (1st) to richest (10th) and the average PISA mathematics score. The OECD averages across all countries tested in 2012 and 2015, as well as England, show a monotonic relationship between wealth and score (Wheater et al., 2016).

Source: NFER analysis of OCED PISA 2012, 2015.

and this is true whether the country does well at maths or not, and whether it is a rich country or not, nor how egalitarian its income or wealth distribution is (see Figure 8.1).

Immigrants

With increasing mobility and with increasing numbers of refugees in European countries, schools have to cope with children from difficult or traumatic backgrounds who may initially be unable to speak the language of the host country. Are these children more likely to have problems learning mathematics? According to the OECD's PISA study, the answer is, on average, no. In fact, they tend to raise the overall level of attainment because, according to Andreas Schleicher, leader of the PISA studies, many migrant families were "hugely motivated" to succeed in education. Of course, there will be challenges where children do not feel they belong, or fail to cope with language and cultural differences (www.bbc.co.uk/news/education-34833547).

There hasn't been, as far as I know, any systematic study of immigrants and dyscalculia.

Language and culture

In the TIMSS survey, children who did not speak the language of the maths test before starting school, did significantly worse on the tests (501 scale points vs 477), though in several countries there was no difference (Mullis et al., 2012; OECD, 2016, Exhibit 4.5).

All the cultures surveyed in TIMSS and PISA are numerate: they have traditional counting practices, and they have sophisticated ways of representing mathematical concepts that have developed over the course of a long history, including our familiar counting words (one, two, three, add, subtract, multiply, equals ...) and our symbols for numbers and their relationships (1, 2, 3, +, -, x, =, etc.). And, they have a system of formal education to teach children about these things. These all help make thinking about and communicating numerical ideas easier (Whitehead, 1948). Nevertheless, there are problems which can be a challenge to the learner: our words for numbers and their relationships have other meanings: "one" can refer to an unspecified person, "two" sounds the same as a word with a different meaning ("too"); "makes", "of", "and", "add" have numerical as well as non-numerical uses. "Three and three *makes* six"; "half *of* six is three"; "*add* milk to the mixture". Even when a numerical meaning is intended, there are several different types of meaning: five cats is more than four cats (cardinal or numerosity meaning), but page 5 isn't more than page 4 (ordinal meaning), but an indication of sequence; *Channel 4* is just a label, and isn't even a sequence (label meaning). Children who fail to make these linguistic distinctions are going to have a hard time learning arithmetic. Unfortunately, there is little or no research on this.

Now, there are still a few small surviving cultures that are not numerate: there are no counting practices, and sometimes not even counting words. These cultures exist in remote regions of Amazonia and of Australia. We have studied children growing up in two such cultures in Australia's Northern Territory: Warlpiri in the Central Desert near Alice Springs and Anindilyakwa on an island off the north coast of Arnhemland. Do these children have normal number concepts? That is, do they have the same concepts of number as we do? According to the inherited core capacity theory (Chapter 3), they should have.

Of course, without counting words, we can't ask these children to say how many objects there are in a display, and we can't ask them even questions that would be straightforwardly understood by children at school in Melbourne, such as "What is three add two?" We had to find another way of doing these tests (see Figure 8.2).

We compared the results on numerosity estimation and non-verbal addition of these Warlpiri and Anindilyakwa children with English-speaking children in schools in Melbourne, and we found very similar performance in both Northern Territory children and those in Melbourne, suggesting that they were both using the same cognitive mechanism, their number module (Butterworth et al., 2008).

Thus, with no cultural support, humans, like many other species, can carry out simple numerical tasks. For more sophisticated arithmetic, learning to use cultural symbols such as counting words and digits, will be very helpful.

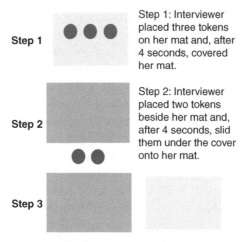

Step 1: Interviewer placed three tokens on her mat and, after 4 seconds, covered her mat.

Step 2: Interviewer placed two tokens beside her mat and, after 4 seconds, slid them under the cover onto her mat.

Step 3: Child attempts to reproduce combined set on child's mat.

Figure 8.2 Non-verbal addition with Anindilyakwa-speaking children. After Steps 1 and 2, the interviewer asked the child to make their mat the same as the interviewer's. For estimation tasks, there is no Step 2: the interviewer's mat is simply covered and the child has to reproduce what was on the mat.

After Butterworth et al., 2008; Reeve et al., 2018.

School

The international surveys reveal many unsurprising results. For example, that poorly-resourced schools do worse (Mullis et al., 2012, Exhibit 5.8); paying teachers poorly reduces average attainment (OECD, 2013, p. 27).

Given the importance of maths to the economy, the UK, among many other countries, has worried that we are not doing as well as we should. From the Cockcroft Report in 1982 on mathematics education onwards, the UK has been concerned at the level of attainment of learners in school. For example, there has been Professor Adrian Smith's report on post-14 maths (Smith, 2004) and Sir Peter Williams' report on primary maths (Williams, 2008). Similarly, the US National Research Council (Council, 2009) noted that "The new demands of international competition in the 21st century require a workforce that is competent in and comfortable with mathematics"; and to that end "The committee [of experts] was charged with examining existing research in order to develop appropriate mathematics learning objectives for preschool children; providing evidence based insights related to curriculum, instruction, and teacher education for achieving these learning objectives" (p. 1). This concern for the general level of mathematics – I will return specifically to numeracy in a moment – is understandable, and in economic terms, justifiable. An OECD modelling exercise showed that the level of maths attainment is a causative factor in long-term economic growth (OECD, 2010).

These reports focused on the standards of teaching and teachers, so for example, Cockcroft required better mathematics education for teachers, and Smith's report recommended the setting up of a National Centre for Excellence in the Teaching of Mathematics (which indeed happened). Improving teaching would, it was implied, improve the average level of attainment. More specifically, a study by the UK's Department for Education and Employment in 1998, which was titled *Numeracy Matters* made a range of recommendations about the teaching of numeracy to raise the average level of attainment (Reynolds, 1998).

These changes are not reflected in a rise in maths attainment at fifteen years (OECD, 2013; 2016) nor in younger children (Mullis et al., 2012). The TIMSS study even suggests that England is going backwards.

Now a national average does not show the range of individual differences in maths attainment. According to the most recent PISA study

> 23% of students in OECD countries, and 32% of students in all participating countries and economies, did not reach the baseline Level 2 in the PISA mathematics assessment of 15 year olds. At that level, students can only extract relevant information from a single source and can use basic algorithms, formulae, procedures or conventions to solve problems involving whole numbers.
> (OECD, 2013, p. 4)

This failure to reach Level 2 varied from 3.8% in Shanghai China to 74.6% in Peru. In the US, it is 25.8%, and in UK it is 21.8%.

These reports did not address the question as to why some learners are stuck at the bottom of the distribution, apart from inadequate access to appropriate teaching. The recently created charity, National Numeracy, aims to raise the standard of numeracy in the UK. Their starting point is "that a major shift in attitudes is key to this." The problem lies with "negative attitudes" (www.nationalnumeracy.org.uk).

One aspect of this is children's motivation to learn maths. Does grouping – or "streaming" – by ability promote motivation? The answer is clear: No it doesn't. Exactly the reverse, in fact (OECD, 2013,)p. 29). See Chapter 11 on policy.

Of course, I argue that in the case of dyscalculia the problem is not negative attitudes but a core deficit in the number module, and as I mentioned in Chapter 1, National Numeracy neglects dyscalculia almost completely, apart from reference to a few books.

Now, all of the reports I have mentioned also neglect dyscalculia, and offer no guidance as to how to identify sufferers or help them progress. What is worse, in the UK, neither Initial Teacher Training (ITT) nor the Postgraduate Certificate in Education (PGCE) in the UK teach teachers about dyscalculia. This means that teachers will not be able to recognise or to help dyscalculics in their class.

There are a few specialist courses available, some just one day, some longer, that teach about dyscalculia.

There is another problem. To be a teacher in the UK you need to attain *Qualified Teacher Status* (QTS). This can be obtained through ITT or PGCE, as well through certain other routes, for example, for graduates or for overseas candidates. In every case, there is a requirement for the candidate to have GCSE maths or its equivalent, a special QTS maths test, and these involve a lot of arithmetic calculations against the clock. This is the case whatever level you are teaching. Many aspiring or experienced teachers fail at this hurdle.

Home

The home environment is shaped by societal factors, and within these, parental education and socio-economic status. Home, school and society, of course, interrelate in many ways. What happens at home, and more specifically in the interactions of the child with parents and carers, turns out to be crucial. But what is it about the home environment that promotes or inhibits the development of arithmetical competence?

According to TIMSS, what happens in the home *before* the child goes to school affects achievement, and not just when the child starts school, but can persist into fourth and even eighth grade and beyond.

> There is increasing evidence that participating in numeracy activities ... during the preschool years can have beneficial effects on children's later acquisition of numeracy skills. To examine students' early home experiences, TIMSS includes an Early Numeracy Activities scale based on parents' reports about the frequency of having done six activities with their child, such as playing with number toys, counting things, and playing number or card games.
>
> (Mullis et al., 2012, p. 11)

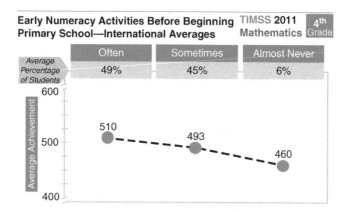

Figure 8.3 The effects of pre-school numerical activities in home.

From Mullis et al., 2012.

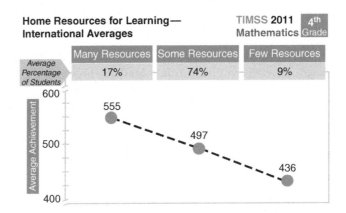

Figure 8.4 The effects of numerical resources in the home on achievement in fourth grade of primary school.

Mullis et al., 2012.

TIMSS also explored the amount of numerical *resources* in the home. These included parents' education, parents' occupation, books in the home, and study supports. Figure 8.4 shows that these had a large effect on achievement in both the fourth and eighth grades.

We tried to look at these factors in more detail in a study of pre-school activities in Italian homes. One potential causal factor is that socially more advantaged parents with better numeracy and higher numeracy expectations engaged in more numeracy-related practices. Was it possible, we asked, to separate the effects of parental education and SES from the actual activities? These numerical activities in the home, though associated with parental education and socio-economic status, have a specific effect over and above these two variables (Benavides-Varela et al., 2016). Our starting point was the pioneering study of Belinda Blevins-Knabe and Linda Musun-Miller who investigated the frequency of specific child and parent child activities at home that directly involved the use of numbers (Blevins-Knabe & Musun-Miller, 1996). The results showed a positive correlation between activities that reflect direct number instruction (i.e. does the child say the words "one", "two", "three", or does the child mention number facts such as 1 + 1 = 2) and children's total scores on standardized tests of early arithmetical ability.

We elaborated their method by using a questionnaire for the parents and one for the child about activities in the home, and cross-checked what they said. We asked about activities used by parents for the explicit purpose of developing numeracy skills, and those where it is incidental, such as board games and some computer games (Skwarchuk et al., 2014) as well as shopping and talking about money with the children, along with more general questions about reading and other games. In addition to the questionnaires, we carried out number sense tests, such as magnitude comparison and a number line task (see Chapter 2 for examples); and we asked questions about numbers in everyday situations, such as, "Could you show me two types of fruits or vegetables that together will make seven pieces?", "Are there fewer lemons or fewer strawberries?"; and money usage, for example, "each one of these vegetables costs one euro. Could you bring me the box that contains the number of vegetables that will make you spend all this money (five euros)?" We looked at the effects of each of these on known precursors of school arithmetic competence: counting, one-to-one correspondence, and everyday numerical problems. The overall frequency of number activities in the home influenced all of these positively, while controlling for socio-economic status.

Summary

- Social, school and home factors all affect the development of numeracy.
- Educational resources and equity affect development
- Numerical activities in the home give children a flying start in school
- None of these factors cause dyscalculia. Even the extreme case of a non-numerate culture, these factors do not cause dyscalculia.

References

Benavides-Varela, S., Butterworth, B., Burgio, F., Arcara, G., Lucangeli, D., & Semenza, C. (2016). Numerical Activities and Information Learned at Home Link to the Exact Numeracy Skills in 5–6 Years-Old Children. *Frontiers in Psychology*, 7(94). doi: 10.3389/fpsyg.2016.00094

Blevins-Knabe, B., & Musun-Miller, L. (1996). Number Use at Home by Children and Their Parents and Its Relationship to Early Mathematical Performance. *Early Development and Parenting*, 5(1), 35–45. doi: 10.1002/(SICI)1099–0917(199603)5:1<35:: AID-EDP113>3.0.CO;2-0

Butterworth, B., Reeve, R., Reynolds, F., & Lloyd, D. (2008). Numerical thought with and without words: Evidence from indigenous Australian children. *Proceedings of the National Academy of Sciences of the USA*, 105, 13179–13184. doi: 10.1073pnas.0806045105

Grantham-McGregor, Sally, Cheung, Yin Bun, Cueto, Santiago, Glewwe, Paul, Richter, Linda, & Strupp, Barbara. (2007). Developmental potential in the first 5 years for children in developing countries. *The Lancet*, 369(9555), 60–70. doi: 10.1016/S0140–6736(07)60032-4

Melhuish, E. C., Sylva, K., Sammons, P., Siraj-Blatchford, I., Taggart, B., Phan, M. B., & Malin, A. (2008). Preschool Influences on Mathematics Achievement. *Science*, 321, 1161–1162.

Mullis, I. V. S., Martin, M. O., Foy, P., & Arora, A. (2012). *TIMSS 2011 International Results in Mathematics*. Chestnut Hill, MA, USA; Amsterdam, the Netherlands. TIMSS & PIRLS International Study Center, Lynch School of Education, Boston College and International Association for the Evaluation of Educational Achievement (IEA) IEA Secretariat. Retrieved from: https://timssandpirls.bc.edu/timss2011/downloads/t11_ir_mathematics_fullbook.pdf

National Research Council. (2009). *Mathematics Learning in Early Childhood: Paths Toward Excellence and Equity.* Washington, DC: National Research Council Center for Education, Division of Behavioral and Social Sciences and Education. Retrieved from: www.nap.edu/catalog/12519/mathematics-learning-in-early-childhood-paths-toward-excellence-and-equity

OECD. (2010). The High Cost of Low Educational Performance. The Long-run Economic Impact of Improving Educational Outcomes. Retrieved from: www.oecd.org/pisa/44417824.pdf

OECD. (2013). PISA 2012 Results in Focus. Retrieved from: www.oecd.org/pisa/keyfindings/pisa-2012-results-overview.pdf

OECD. (2016). PISA 2015 Results in Focus. Retrieved from: www.oecd.org/pisa/pisa-2015-results-in-focus.pdf

Reeve, R. A., Reynolds, F., Paul, J., & Butterworth, B. L. (2018). Culture-Independent Prerequisites for Early Arithmetic. *Psychological Science*, 0956797618769893. doi: 10.1177/0956797618769893

Reynolds, D. (1998). *Numeracy Matters: The Preliminary Report of the Numeracy Task Force* (1998). London: Department for Education and Employment.

Shaw, B., Bernardes, E., Trethewey, A., & Menzies, L. (2016). *Special educational needs and their links to poverty.* Joseph Rowntree Foundation.

Shaw, P., Greenstein, D., Lerch, J., Clasen, L., Lenroot, R., Gogtay, N., Evans, A., Rapoport, J., & Giedd, J. (2006). Intellectual ability and cortical development in children and adolescents. *Nature*, 440(7084), 676–679. doi: 10.1038/nature04513

Skwarchuk, Sheri-Lynn, Sowinski, Carla, & LeFevre, Jo-Anne. (2014). Formal and informal home learning activities in relation to children's early numeracy and literacy skills: The development of a home numeracy model. *Journal of Experimental Child Psychology*, 121, 63–84. doi: 10.1016/j.jecp.2013.11.006

Smith, A. (2004). *Making Mathematics Count: The Report of Professor Adrian Smith's Inquiry into Post-14 Mathematics Education* (Vol. 937764). London: The Stationery Office Limited.

Wheater, R., Durbin, B., McNamara, S., & Classick, R. (2016). Is mathematics education in England working for everyone? NFER analysis of the PISA performance of disadvantaged pupils. Retrieved from: www.nfer.ac.uk/is-mathematics-education-in-england-working-for-everyone-nfer-analysis-of-the-pisa-performance-of-disadvantaged-pupils/

Whitehead, A. N. (1948). *An Introduction to Mathematics* (originally published in 1911). London: Oxford University Press.

Williams, P. (2008). Independent Review of Mathematics Teaching in Early Years Settings and Primary Schools: Final Report. (DCSF-00433–2008).

Assessment

How to identify dyscalculic learners

LEVEL OF EXPLANATION	MEASURES	EDUCATIONAL CONTEXT
BEHAVIOURAL	Number sense Chapter 2	Society, school and home Chapter 8
COGNITIVE	Starter kit for learning arithmetic Chapter 3 Core deficit as the cause of dyscalculia Chapter 4	**Assessment Chapter 9** Intervention Chapter 10 Policy Chapter 11
	Development of arithmetic Chapter 5	
NEURAL	Brain structures and functions Chapter 6	
GENETIC AND OTHER CAUSES Chapter 7		

Purposes of assessment

The first thing the assessor has to decide is why this assessment is being made. This might seem like a redundant question, since it is obvious that the person being assessed is not doing as well as expected. However, the reason for the assessment will shape how to do the assessment.

There are two main reasons for doing an assessment:

1. *Assessment for support.* To see whether someone is entitled for special help or special "accommodations" in exams or at work.
2. *Assessment for intervention.* To evaluate cognitive strengths and weaknesses in order to design the appropriate intervention strategy.

In addition to these reasons, many sufferers, parents or teachers simply want know why the child is failing. This will help them to resolve concerns that a struggling individual and his or her connections have about the causes of the difficulty. Learners need to know that their failures can be quite specific: they are not simply stupid or lazy or naughty. Parents also need to know this, and teachers need to know that a learner's lack of progress is not due to their own incompetence as teachers (see Chapter 10 for more on intervention).

Each of these reasons implies different tests and different assessments. (As is often said, tests test, but people assess.) In this chapter, I try to lay out the basic principles for assessment with illustrative examples. Bear in mind that the rules and regulations may, and often do, change.

Assessment for support

Which kind of assessment is undertaken will depend on the laws and regulations set down by the relevant authorities. I described these in some detail in Chapter 1.

UK

The Children and Families Act of 2014 defines children with special educational needs or disability (SEND) as having "a significantly greater difficulty in learning than the majority of others of the same age". It requires that "'Special educational provision', for a child aged two or more or a young person, means educational or training provision that is additional to, or different from, that made generally for others of the same age." This should lead to additional resources being made available to the school for the special educational provision. The SEND learner should get an education, health and care (EHC) plan for children and young people who need more support than is available through special educational needs support. The local authority decides whether a child deserves an EHC, but once an EHC plan has been issued, the education provision has to be provided. Exactly how the local authority agrees to this is complicated, and seems to depend on its procedures and, presumably, the straitened state of its finances.

With some exceptions (e.g. children diagnosed with autism), schools do not receive direct funds for children with special learning needs. Schools, however, may assign funds to specialist teachers (e.g. reading specialists) from their own budget. In addition, schools most often refer children with learning difficulties, including mathematics learning difficulty (MLD), to a State-funded educational psychologist, attached to the school or groups of schools in an area.

However, dyscalculia, as distinct from other causes of MLD, is not specifically covered in the regulations on provision for SEND learners. Dyscalculia is not referred to in UK law nor on the UK Department for Education website, except insofar as it is not a bar to a driving license for cars and motor cycles, but it is a bar to driving heavy vehicles such as busses and lorries. Nevertheless, or perhaps because of the lack of governmental specificity, several bodies have taken on the task of defining dyscalculia and recommending procedures for assessing it.

British Dyslexia Association

Perhaps the most visible and important of these bodies is British Dyslexia Association, which now recognizes dyscalculia as a distinct SpLD (Specific Learning Difficulty), and has set up a dyscalculia committee on which I sit. The BDA defines dyscalculia as

> a specific learning disorder that is characterised by impairments in learning basic arithmetic facts, processing numerical magnitude and performing accurate and fluent calculations. These difficulties must be quantifiably below what is expected for an individual's chronological age, and must not be caused by poor educational or daily activities or by intellectual impairments.
>
> (www.bdadyslexia.org.uk/dyslexic/dyscalculia)

An internal document that is incorporated into BDA accredited courses (see below) lays out a scheme for assessment which distinguishes dyscalculia from other causes of maths learning difficulty or disability:

> For the purposes of diagnostic assessment, it is recommended that 5 conditions be considered. The first 4 conditions must be present for a diagnosis of maths learning difficulty, and all five for a diagnosis of dyscalculia:

1. There is a past history of maths difficulties
2. There is evidence that maths difficulties are currently impacting negatively on academic performance, and/or employment, and/or every-day life.
3. The test score for a standardised maths test is significantly lower than expected for the age/experience of the child/student/adult.
4. A low score on a test of maths is not due solely to inappropriate teaching, poor mathematical memory, slow speed of working or impoverished experience when young/before school.

> A diagnosis of dyscalculia can be considered when the above conditions are satisfied **PLUS**:

5. There is a deficit in understanding simple number concepts, lacking an intuitive grasp of numbers, which can show itself in estimating the number of objects in a set.

This criterion is taken from a DfES document (UK ministry of education in 2001, but is no longer included in the current UK government's guidelines, since it no longer recognizes dyscalculia – see Chapter 1). It also corresponds to the position taken in this book, that dyscalculia is a core deficit in the "number module" – an inherited neural mechanism that underpins basic numerical processing (see especially Chapters 3 and 4).

SASC (SpLD Assessment and Standards Committee)

This is a non-governmental association to which the BDA and other bodies are affiliated, and which endorses assessment procedure and courses for professionals working with SpLD. Although the procedure they recommend has similarities with that proposed by the BDA, there are important differences:

■ A diagnosis of dyscalculia depends on there being a discrepancy between performance on a standardized maths test and IQ. This is similar to the discrepancy criterion used in DSM-IV (see Chapter 1).

SASC does not require that there is *a deficit in understanding simple number concepts, lacking an intuitive grasp of numbers, which can show itself in estimating the number of objects in a set.*

SASC does provide detailed advice for assessing older dyscalculics, particularly students at institutes of higher education.

It is important to make a clear distinction between students whose mathematical difficulties are due to dyslexia or other neurodiversities and those who struggle with mathematics as a result of dyscalculia. Consideration must be given to the other possible factors such as knowledge gaps through poor teaching, long periods of absence or mathematical anxiety. Problems learning number facts and procedures could be due to a reliance on rote learning and recall, areas known to be at risk for dyslexic people.

"Dyscalculia is a condition that affects the ability to acquire arithmetical skills. Dyscalculic learners may have difficulty understanding simple number concepts, lack an intuitive grasp of numbers, and have problems learning number facts and procedures. Even if they produce a correct answer or use a correct method, they may do so mechanically and without confidence" (The National Numeracy Strategy (DfES (2001)).

Initial screening is a useful indicator, although currently, few tests exist for the post 16 population. DysCalculiUM [see below Online Tests] is a first-line computer-based screening tool, developed by Trott and Beacham, and is designed to focus on the fundamental understanding of mathematics. The resulting profile provides an indication of "at risk" for 11 categories based on number and their applications. This is not sufficient on its own, however, as a diagnostic tool.

The following is recommended in an assessment for dyscalculia:

1. Initial screening test for dyscalculia
2. A full assessment of verbal and non-verbal cognitive abilities (including matrices); compare non-verbal reasoning with age expectation and verbal reasoning and standardised test of mathematical ability

3. A standardised test of mathematical ability compared with age expectation: a. Compare with age expectation; b. Compare with intelligence; c. Compare with verbal reasoning
4. A full personal history, particularly with regard to mathematics. This should include mathematical experiences through school and how the student manages with everyday situations in which number/mathematics are used.
5. Observed test behaviour for indications of mathematical anxiety or tension and lack of confidence in tackling mathematical calculations and problems.

(http://bit.ly/2BcMCCS)

JCQ (Joint Council for Qualifications)

This is a membership organization comprising the seven largest providers of qualifications in the UK. It is not a government body, and it includes for profit companies, such as Pearson. It can authorize "Adjustments for candidates with disabilities and learning difficulties" including dyscalculia. Their regulations state:

Candidates with learning difficulties may require for example: supervised rest breaks [and] extra time [in exams].

However, most of the adjustments under this heading are for learners with dyslexia.

(http://bit.ly/2s7ZS9a)

Australia

There is no official – federal government – definition of dyscalculia, or even maths learning difficulty or disability (MLD), despite the fact that learning pathways in primary school are laid out in detail with only minor local variations. Each state seems to have its own approach to MLD.

In a review of provisions for dyscalculia and MLD in Australia, my Melbourne University colleague, Robert Reeve, writes

The Federal Government's Senate Education and Employment References Committee Report (2016) discussion on the needs of students with LD highlights this point (even though MLD is not mentioned explicitly).

One dimension of the problems with data ... is that current funding models have failed to adequately fund the education of students with disability because they have taken too narrow a definition of disability. If a student's disability is not recognised as such in the funding model, that model clearly cannot provide the financial assistance necessary to properly assist that child's access to education.

Due to the inadequate support in the current school environment families are required to repeatedly advocate for their child's needs. This is particularly true for students who do not qualify for a diagnosis of intellectual disability (or any of the other specific funding categories) and hence must attend mainstream classes without teacher's aide support. The impact of this in practical terms is that even if an IEP (Individual Education Plan) is formulated by the school based on the child's individual needs, recommendations are not always able to be implemented due to lack of support staff. The end result is a maintenance or worsening of the child's behaviour and a stagnation of the learning process, resulting in unsatisfactory outcomes for all.

The committee was concerned by evidence suggesting that many students have fallen through funding cracks because of limited information or narrow definitions of disability used in school systems, resulting in a failure to recognise need. An appropriate level of funding for students with additional needs in schools begins with adequate data on those students.

(Reeve, in press)

By contrast with official neglect, and rather like the BDA in the UK, AUSPELD, an independent organization which supports people with learning disabilities nationwide, recognizes dyscalculia as a specific learning disability.

The Dyslexia SPELD Foundation in Perth, Western Australia, lays out their approach very clearly. Here I follow Mandy Nayton, their Chief Executive Officer and Kelly Fullarton, their senior psychologist. The diagnosis of dyscalculia is based on DSM-5 (see Chapter 1) that emphasizes *persistent failure to respond to intervention, and the exclusion of other possible explanations*. This means that it may be possible to recognize dyscalculia in children in the first year of school and even earlier, since teaching, especially special teaching, can count as an intervention.

The case of Sally

Kelly Fullarton, in a lecture to educational psychologists in 2015, illustrated this approach in relation to a case study of one learner, Sally:

- 7 Years 5 months of age. Currently in Year 3. Developmental history unremarkable. Hearing and vision tested within normal range. Has consistently attended school and is a well-regarded student with no behavioural issues. No concerns noted in Kindergarten and Pre-Primary.
- Literacy and numeracy delays first noted in Year 1 and she was provided with school-based support across both areas. Positive response to literacy interventions (now within the range of her peers) but continues to be underperforming in numeracy. Private tuition for 18 months with

a focus on early number and arithmetic skills. Referred for diagnostic testing by the classroom teacher.

Using the DSM-5 approach requires satisfying all four diagnostic criteria:

1. Difficulties learning and using academic skills that have persisted for at least 6 months despite the provision of intervention that targets those difficulties.
   (a) Sally failed to make satisfactory response to intervention despite curriculum-based support at school for >12 months, and skills-based specialist intervention for 18 months.
   (b) Therefore, numeracy delays are considered *persistent*
2. The affected academic skills are substantially and quantifiably below those expected based on chronological age, AND cause significant interference with academic or occupational performance.
   (c) These can be based on standardized assessment tools of calculation fluency and numbers sense, such as the WIAT, Woodcock Johnson, TEMA, and the Dyscalculia Screener.
   (d) Sally remained below average for her age on number sense and calculation tests, but her non-numerical cognitive tests were in the average range.
3. The learning difficulties begin during school-age years but may not become apparent until the demands of those affected academic skills exceed the individual's limited capacities (e.g. timed tests and heavy study loads)
   (e) Sally is currently of school age and has experienced persistent numeracy difficulties throughout her education.
4. The learning difficulties are not better accounted for by intellectual disabilities, uncorrected hearing and vision difficulties, other mental or neurological disorders, psychosocial adversity, lack of proficiency in the language of instruction or inadequate education experience.
   (f) Sally is of average range intellectual ability.
   (g) Her hearing and vision are within the normal limits
   (h) She does not present with a mental or neurological disorder.
   (i) Sally has attended school consistently and appropriate numeracy teaching has been in place.
   (j) There are no language delays

Therefore, there are no other factors that would better account for Sally's ongoing numeracy delays. Therefore, Sally has a specific deficit in numerical abilities or dyscalculia.

USA

The Individuals with Disabilities Education Act (IDEA) in USA recognizes dyscalculia (along with dyslexia), as I mentioned in Chapter 1.

The Office of Special Education and Rehabilitative Services of the USA's Department of Education requires state and local education authorities to carry out appropriate assessments and to provide appropriate help.

> The Office of Special Education Programs (OSEP) funds a large network of technical assistance centers that develop materials and resources to support States, school districts, schools, and teachers to improve the provision of services to children with disabilities, including materials on the use of accommodations … [which refers] to the various components of a free appropriate public education, including special education, related services, supplementary aids and services, and program modifications or supports for school personnel, as well as accommodations for students taking assessments.
>
> (Yudin, 2015)

"All children with disabilities … who are in need of special education and related services, are identified, located and evaluated" (Section 612(a)(3) of IDEA). This can, and presumably should, lead to an Individual Education Plan. There is also a legal duty to ensure that the provision required in the Plan is made available to the child, and to monitor progress on a regular basis.

In addition to the provisions in IDEA, insurance may cover some of the costs of assessment and support. For this, reference to "bibles" such as DSM 5 and ICD 10 is required. ICD 10 uses the term "specific disorder of arithmetical skills … that is not solely explicable on the basis of general mental retardation or of inadequate schooling." A *billable* ICD-10-CM code can be used to indicate a diagnosis for reimbursement purposes. However, neither DSM 5 nor ICD 10 state or recommend a particular test battery, nor the criterion for specific disorder of arithmetical skills.

Who is qualified to make an assessment of dyscalculia?

In the UK, it could be the teacher who notices that a child is not responding to teaching and is falling further and further behind classmates. All children in state schools take exams (SATS – Statutory Assessment Tests) in their second year – about seven years old, this could provide the teacher or parent with information about learners who are falling behind. It would be better, though, if the learner could be identified in the first year.

For the learner falling behind, the teacher can initiate steps to find specialist support or an EHCP. Sometimes, it will be a worried parent who initiates these steps. This will typically involve the school's SENCO (Special Educational

Needs Coordinator) who can refer the child to an educational psychologist or other qualified professional for an assessment. However, not all schools have a SENCO, including many private schools and schools outside local educational authority control.

Assuming that a formal assessment is requested, the question arises as to who is qualified to carry it out. Unfortunately, it is rare for teachers or psychologists to receive training to assess dyscalculia. In my experience of teaching on teacher training, educational psychologist post-graduate courses and continuing professional development courses, fewer than half had even heard of dyscalculia prior to the course.

In the UK, as I have noted, dyscalculia is not recognized by government bodies, and it falls upon the SASC (SpLD Assessment and Standards Committee) to oversee and approve processes of awarding SpLD Assessment Practising Certificates. There are currently three awarding bodies for SpLD Assessment Practising Certificates for specialist teachers. The BDA, PATOSS and the Dyslexia Guild (with Dyslexia Action as its training arm).

AMBDA [Associate Membership of the BDA] would qualify for appropriate membership of an SpLD Assessment Practising Certificate.

PATOSS is "[t]he professional association of teachers of students with specific learning difficulties". It deals in depth and at length with dyslexia (its email is info@patoss-dyslexia), and almost nothing on dyscalculia.

Dyslexia Action offers "specialist teacher training accredited by the British Dyslexia Association (BDA) and by the SpLD Assessment Standards Committee (SASC)". It offers a short course at Level 4 for teachers and teaching assistants, but this is not a qualification to assess for dyscalculia.

What all this means is that it is still very hard to find qualified person, usually a clinical, occupational or educational psychologist, who has had either the training or the experience to make a proper assessment.

There are nevertheless specialist centres with extensive experience of dyscalculia. One that I have worked with is Emerson House, co-founded by Jane Emerson and Dorian Yeo (see above). Some universities have dedicated centres for their students with special learning needs, such as Mathematics Education Centre at Loughborough University where Clare Trott has a track record of identifying students with dyscalculia and helping them.

A few post-graduate courses on SpLD are now beginning to include dyscalculia.

Tests

Psychologists will use a range of tests with norms based on samples of children which can give an indication of how the child compares with other children of their own age. This will require a decision about the point at which the child is significantly different from peers, and this is essentially an arbitrary point in terms of percentiles (e.g. the lowest 10%) or in terms of standard deviation units.

Psychological batteries such the WIAT II (Wechsler Individual Achievement Test for Teachers) or the British Abilities Scale enable the assessor to compare performance on the maths subtests with tests of general cognitive ability. DSM IV requires a significant discrepancy between the maths level and the IQ level for a diagnosis of mathematics learning disability (though note that DSM 5 does not, see above and Chapter 1). However, these tests do not distinguish dyscalculia from other causes of mathematics disability apart from those attributable to general cognitive problems.

Various organizations and individuals offer checklists of symptoms of dyscalculia that may occur in everyday life, such as:

- Inconsistent results in addition, subtraction, multiplication and division.
- Bad at financial planning and money management.
- Too slow at mental math to figure totals, change due, tip, tax.
- Difficulty keeping track of time.
- Frequently late.

They often include symptoms that may or may not have anything to do with numerical ability, such as:

- Mistaken recollection of names.
- Poor name–face association.
- Substitute names beginning with same letter.

In my view, a checklist at best is an indicator that a proper assessment is needed.

Feifer Assessment of Mathematics

This is "a comprehensive tests of mathematics designed to examine the underlying neurodevelopmental processes that support the acquisition of proficient math skills". It uses paper and pencil tests with time limits, and has been standardized on a large cohort of US participants, age graded. It provides three indices:

- The Verbal Index score is a measure of automatic fact retrieval and the linguistic components of math.
- The Procedural Index score is a measure of a student's ability to count, order, and sequence numbers or mathematical procedures.
- The Semantic Index score is a measure of visual–spatial and conceptual components, including magnitude representation, patterns and relationships, higher-level mathematical problem solving, and number sense. This includes digit comparison.

As far as I can tell, there are no peer-reviewed reports of the validity or reliability of this test. It costs US$502 for ten examinations (http://bit.ly/2ENshUv).

Digital tests

Several online tests are currently available specifically for assessing dyscalculia in children and adults.

CogniFit

This describes itself as an "[i]nnovative neuropsychological assessment for dyscalculia that allows for a complete cognitive screening and assessment of the risk index of having this math-based learning disorder with excellent reliability". The website references only the effects of cognitive training with the elderly, but not validity or reliability of the method. Costs £49.95 (http://bit.ly/2C1DEW3).

The Dyscalculia Test – teachers

This has been developed by Tony Attwood, an experienced dyscalculia professional. It is untimed which is a limitation, since the time taken to do numerical tasks is diagnostic, as I have argued at length in this book. It is not clear whether there is evidence of the reliability or validity of this test. When the test has been completed, a report will be sent. Costs £59.95 (http://bit.ly/2nJaEOy).

Numeracy Screener

This has been developed in the lab of Daniel Ansari, a leading expert in the brain and numerical cognition. It is based on two tests: comparing the magnitude of two dot arrays and comparing the magnitude of two digits. Ansari and colleagues have presented extensive peer-reviewed evidence that these tests, especially the digit test, correlate with arithmetical ability. The test is not item-timed, but depends on the number of items completed within a time limit. However, they also point out that

> The numeracy screener is not a diagnostic tool. It cannot be used to tell whether a child has a specific learning difficulty in the domain of numeracy and mathematics, such as Developmental Dyscalculia. It is meant as a screener for potential strengths and weaknesses among students. The Numeracy Screener is merely one of many tests that can inform teachers, parents and educational psychologists about the numerical processing abilities of a child. Put differently, a low score on the numeracy screener may serve to alert a parent, teacher, psychologist to carry out additional testing.

It's free (http://bit.ly/2C1HI8L).

Panamath

This was developed at Johns Hopkins University by Justin Halberda and his colleagues to test "number sense" (see Chapter 2). It has been extensively evaluated and reported in peer-reviewed publications. It shows that there is a reasonable correlation between the ability to select the larger number of dots and arithmetical competence. Performance is age-related, and they present age-appropriate data. Poor performance may be an indicator that proper assessment is needed but this test in itself is not a test for dyscalculia. It's free (www.panamath.org/index.php).

The Dyscalculia Screener

This screener is for dyscalculia based on the approach taken in this book. It has been standardised on a UK population of six- to 14-year-olds. It includes two tests of *core capacity* – dot enumeration and digit comparison, and an item-timed test of single-digit addition and, for older testees, single-digit multiplication. The learner must score in the lowest 7% on the capacity tests to count as dyscalculic. The software generates both a description of the data and a narrative that distinguishes dyscalculics from those who are bad at the arithmetic tests but are normal on the capacity tests. There is extensive evidence that this approach is valid and reliable (Chapter 4). Costs £6.10 per testee (http://bit.ly/2BersnT). (Full disclosure: I get a commission for every sale.)

Dyscalculia-Screener

This is different from the Dyscalculia Screener (above) in that it is for over 16s and appears not to be standardized. It has been developed by a different company, iansyst, and based on different principles.

> The Dyscalculia Screener provides a first step in the process of the identification of dyscalculia for young people and adults. Extensive research has been conducted to develop a range of exercises which, once completed, will provide an instant result based on an overall percentage.... The Dyscalculia Screener is based on a model which is built on two principal objectives: firstly, to establish the learner's understanding of number and, secondly, their understanding of the application of number to other systems. The model outlines six key areas.

The subtests are not described on the website, and it is not clear what criteria are used to determine whether the testee is dyscalculic. I haven't seen any published data on reliability or validity. Costs £30 per testee (http://bit.ly/2C1PeAv).

Assessment for intervention

Here I follow the work of Dorian Yeo, and her colleagues Jane Emerson and Patricia Babtie. In my book with Dorian, the focus was on intervention rather than assessment (Butterworth & Yeo, 2004). Emerson and Babtie, following Dorian, use their own systematic assessment system to inform *teaching plans* for individual learners (Emerson & Babtie, 2013; 2014). They start with an assessment of core capacity – "number sense" – and relevant domain-general cognitive capacities, such as memory and sequencing, as well as the problem of co-occurring development issues in language, reading, attention and anxiety.

The assessment will start with number sense. There will be informal tests of subitizing up to four counters, estimating up to 20 counters, oral counting, reading and writing numbers. Counting skills are particularly informative for early learners because it reflects the underlying understanding of numbers, and forms the conceptual basis of arithmetic (Fuson, 1988; Gelman & Gallistel, 1978) and Chapter 3.

Emerson and Babtie link the outcome of these assessments to *teaching plans*. For example, if the learner has problems in the small numbers of counters, the teaching plan should include practice with dice patterns and encourage recognizing numerosities rather than counting in ones, an almost universal dyscalculic strategy. They also recommend quickly covering the display of objects to promote recognition rather than counting. If there is difficulty with larger numerosities, the plan will include games where random displays of counters should be grouped into sets of tens and then the whole lot counted. This helps with both estimating and the conventional ten-based system.

Dyscalculics may well have acquired some knowledge of more advanced numerical concepts, such as the ten-based place value system, but these may be shaky or incomplete. Further assessments and teaching plans will be required.

The problem of co-morbidity

Emerson and Babtie, as experienced special needs teachers, are well aware that developmental disabilities in addition to dyscalculia are frequent, and need to be assessed separately, and, where necessary, lead to separate interventions.

One commonly co-occurring disability is dyslexia. The British Dyslexia Association notes that "Developmental Dyscalculia often occurs in association with other developmental disorders such as dyslexia or ADHD/ADD" (www.bdadyslexia.org.uk/dyslexic/dyscalculia). It goes on to say that "[c]o-occurrence of learning disorders appears to be the rule rather than the exception". This is at best an exaggeration.

Let us take standard definitions of these neurodevelopmental conditions in Table 9.1.

Now, it is true that co-occurrence, sometimes called "co-morbidity", is much higher than would be expected by chance. Estimates of the prevalence of the relevant neurodevelopmental disorders is given in Table 9.2.

It turns out that the co-occurrence of any of the two conditions in Table 9.2 is statistically highly significant. To take one example, dyslexia and dyscalculia : assume dyslexia has a prevalence of 7%, and dyscalculia a prevalence of 6%, then by chance 6% of dyslexics should also be dyscalculia. Co-occurrences should be very rare as 6% of 7% is 0.42%. However, one population-based study, with these prevalences, found that 23–49% of children in Grades 2 to 4 had disabilities of both literacy and numeracy (Landerl & Moll, 2010). Even with this very significant co-occurrence, there would still be more dyscalculics who are *not* dyslexic than who are, and more dyslexics who are not dyscalculic than who are. Indeed, the most dyslexic person I have ever tested, Dr Kalvis Jansons, who has written about his condition, is a distinguished mathematician. Thus, research shows that co-occurrence is not the *rule* for dyslexia and dyscalculia.

Table 9.1 Definitions of specific learning deficits.

Specific learning disability	Definitions
Developmental dyslexia	Developmental disorder in learning to read not due to impairments in general intelligence, sensory problems, emotional disturbances or inadequate schooling.
Developmental dyscalculia	Substantial underachievement on a standardized test of arithmetic relative to the level expected given age, education, and intelligence which causes disruption to academic achievement or daily living.
Attention-deficit/ hyperactivity disorder	Symptoms of inattention, hyperactivity, impulsivity, such that these symptoms cause clinically significant distress or impairment in social, academic, or occupational functioning.
Autism spectrum disorder	Impairments of social interaction, communication, and repetitive, stereotyped behaviour.
Specific language impairment	Significant deficits in expressive or receptive language, not due to sensory or environmental deprivation, co-occur with non-verbal intelligence within the average range

Adapted from DSM-IV (Diagnostic and Statistical Manual of Mental Disorders of the American Psychiatric Association, Fourth Edition) and/or ICD 10 (International Classification of Diseases, Tenth Edition, of the World Health Organization).

Table 9.2 Estimated prevalences of five Specific Learning Difficulties 2000–2009.

Specific learning difficulty	Estimated prevalence (%)
Dyslexia	4–8
Dyscalculia	3.5–6.5
Attention-deficit/hyperactivity disorder (ADHD)	3–6
Autism spectrum disorder (ASD)	1
Specific language impairment (SLI)	7

From Bishop, 2010; Butterworth & Kovas, 2013.

However, the co-occurrence rate still needs to be explained. In a recent study, that is exactly what we tried to do (Butterworth & Kovas, 2013). We looked at three possible types of explanation: cognitive, neural and genetic. I'll briefly review these before addressing the implications for assessment.

Cognitive factors in co-occurring specific learning difficulties (SpLDs)

Domain-general explanations

The BDA paper notes that "[c]o-occurrence is generally assumed to be a consequence of risk factors that are shared between disorders, for example, working memory". Now, measures of working memory include tests of the ability to reproduce a string of digits in the presented order, while other tasks tap the ability to modify the contents of memory. Although dyslexia is associated with somewhat poorer ability to repeat back a series of words or numbers, the picture for the other SpLDs is much less clear, and depends on the working memory task employed. In fact, SpLDs may actually cause poor performance on some IQ tests. This is most obvious where the IQ test depends on reading and understanding and also a reasonable degree of numeracy. In Chapter 5, I argued that impairments of working memory, intelligence, or processing speed, do not cause dyscalculia, though they may reduce performance on tests of mathematical competence.

Another approach is that these other conditions actually *cause* dyscalculia. The problem here is that the other conditions in Table 9.1 are better known and usually more obvious than dyscalculia because they affect everyday life in ways that teachers and parents notice. This means that children are more likely to be referred for dyslexia, ADHD, autism or SLI (Specific Language Impairment), and therefore, we suggest "[i]t is likely that an unassessed SpLD will be treated as the *consequence* of the assessed SpLD."

Kovas and I argue, on the basis of extensive research, that each of these conditions is due to specific *core cognitive deficits* that are quite different from the core deficit underlying dyscalculia.

> *Dyslexia:* the majority of children diagnosed, have a *phonological deficit* (Snowling, 2000).
> *ADHD:* Children diagnosed with ADHD may have several core cognitive deficits, including one in attention and one in controlling, and especially inhibiting, behaviour.
> *ASD:* A core deficit in representing one's own and other people's thoughts and feelings is implicated in this condition, which is sometimes called a deficit in the "theory of mind" (Baron-Cohen et al., 1985).
> *SLI:* Results from several core deficits, including the phonological deficit that is shared with dyslexia, and also deficits in syntax and word meanings (Bishop & Snowling, 2004).

Neural

There does not seem to be a neural system that is common to any of these conditions and the specific neural abnormalities of dyscalculia I outlined in Chapter 6 that focused on the parietal lobes and in particular the *Intraparietal sulcus* bilaterally. Table 9.3 reports the main structural differences in the SpLDs

Table 9.3 Typical results for structural brain imaging where probands (affected individuals) with a Specific Learning Disability differ significantly from controls. (GMD: Grey Matter Density; WM: White Matter.)

	Structural differences between typically developing and atypically developing	**Source**
Dyslexia	Decreased GMD in left inferior temporal gyri; decreased GMD (grey matter density) in left middle temporal gyri; decreased WM (white matter) in left arcuate fasciculus	(Silani et al., 2005)
Attention-deficit/ hyperactivity disorder	Decreased overall brain volume and cortical thickness; decreased volume of anterior cingulate cortex; decreased frontal cortex volume; basal ganglia, limbic system, cerebellum	(Krain & Castellanos, 2006; Makris et al., 2010; Proal et al., 2011)
Autism spectrum disorder	Greater total brain volume and grey matter volume throughout lifespan, most prominently in frontal lobe; Greater pre-puberty WM volume	(Amaral, Schumann, & Nordahl, 2008)
Specific language impairment	Abnormal perisylvian asymmetry, including left perisylvian volume (abnormal asymmetry)	(Jernigan et al., 1991) (Soriano-Mas et al., 2009)
Dyscalculia	Decreased GMD in left intraparietal sulcus	(Isaacs et al., 2001)

Adapted from Butterworth & Kovas, 2013.

Genetic

Although dyscalculia appears to be congenital – present at birth – this doesn't mean that it is always inherited, as I discussed in Chapter 7. Research currently suggests that all cognitive traits are polygenic – influenced by many genes with small effects, and therefore dyscalculia may be affected by many genes. There is also "pleiotropy" – that is, the same genes may affect multiple traits implicated in different cognitive processes.

Twin studies suggest that the same genes probably affect the diverse neurocognitive processes that underpin all school performance. Twin studies also suggest moderate to substantial genetic correlations (the extent to which the same genes affect different conditions) for ADHD (especially inattention) and Reading/

Mathematics; Autistic Spectrum Disorder and ADHD/Language; Reading, Language, and Mathematics delay.

However, a substantial proportion of genetic variance is linked with a single cognitive domain. For example, in one large twin study of 7 year olds, some 30% of genetic variance was specific to mathematics (Kovas et al., 2007). This finding has been replicated in other studies.

DNA markers – gene variants – associated with cognition and behaviour have a very small effect on any trait, and seem to work throughout the distribution, explaining variation in the normal range, as well as discriminating affected individuals from the unaffected population. There have been recent suggestions that some markers are implicated in both reading and mathematics, but the causal pathway is still unclear.

Implications of co-occurring SpLDs for assessment

Although these disabilities are congenital, they are rarely identified until relatively late in childhood, if at all, and, as we have seen, teachers, parents and even professionals, such as educational psychologists, are often poorly informed about dyscalculia.

If, as I suggested above, the assessed condition is assumed to cause the unassessed condition, this could have serious consequences for learners, their teachers and parents.

For example, if a dyscalculic child is assessed with attention-deficit/hyperactivity disorder, then the maths disability could be assumed to result from that condition, therefore be treated pharmaceutically (e.g. with methylphenidate) but without the specialized help learners with dyscalculia need.

Similarly, a child assessed with dyslexia who also has dyscalculia, may get a learning programme designed to treat the reading disability.

The recommendation therefore is to assess each symptom separately. That is, if the learner has dyslexia and a maths difficulty, assess both to check for a co-occurring dyscalculia, and then use the outcome of the assessment to design the appropriate interventions.

Summary

- The main purposes of assessment:
  - *Assessment for support* which depends on local or national rules and regulations
  - *Assessment for intervention* requires systematic review of the learner's strengths and weaknesses in the number domain
- Methods of assessment
  - Should distinguish dyscalculia from other causes of low attainment
  - Criteria from standardized tests of arithmetic will not identify dyscalculics

- Persistent failure to respond to intervention (DSM 5) is a useful way of identifying children at risk
- Dyscalculic-specific tests, such as the Dyscalculia Screener, will test for a *core deficit*
- The problem of co-morbidity
  - Dyscalculia co-occurs with other neurodevelopmental disabilities much more often than would be expected by chance
  - Since dyscalculia is less well known than dyslexia, ADHD or autism, the dyscalculic learner may be referred for these conditions which are often assumed to be the cause of arithmetical difficulties.
  - There is no known common cognitive, neural or genetic cause of all these conditions, therefore
  - Dyscalculia needs to be assessed separately, and interventions designed specifically

References

Amaral, D. G., Schumann, C. M., & Nordahl, C. W. (2008). Neuroanatomy of autism. *Trends Neurosci*, 31(3), 137–145. doi: 10.1016/j.tins.2007.12.005

Baron-Cohen, S., Leslie, A. M., & Frith, U. (1985). Does the autistic child have a "theory of mind"? *Cognition*, 21(1), 37–46. doi: 10.1016/0010–0277(85)90022-8

Bishop, D. V. M. (2010). Which Neurodevelopmental Disorders Get Researched and Why? *PLoS ONE*, 5(11): e15112. doi: 10.1371/journal.pone.0015112

Bishop, D. V. M., & Snowling, M. (2004). Developmental Dyslexia and Specific Language Impairment: Same or Different? *Psychological Bulletin*, 130, 858–886.

Butterworth, B., & Kovas, Y. (2013). Understanding Neurocognitive Developmental Disorders Can Improve Education for All. *Science*, 340(6130), 300–305. doi: 10.1126/science.1231022

Butterworth, B., & Yeo, D. (2004). *Dyscalculia Guidance*. London: nferNelson.

Emerson, J., & Babtie, P. (2013). *The Dyscalculia Assessment* (Second edition). London: Bloomsbury Education.

Emerson, J., & Babtie, P. (2014). *The Dyscalculia Solution: Teaching Number Sense*. London: Bloomsbury Education.

Fuson, K. C. (1988). *Children's Counting and Concepts of Number*. New York: Springer Verlag.

Gelman, R., & Gallistel, C. R. (1978). *The Child's Understanding of Number* (1986 edition). Cambridge, MA: Harvard University Press.

Isaacs, E. B., Edmonds, C. J., Lucas, A., & Gadian, D. G. (2001). Calculation difficulties in children of very low birthweight: A neural correlate. *Brain*, 124, 1701–1707.

Jernigan, T. L., Hesselink, J. R., Sowell, E., & Tallal, P. A. (1991). Cerebral structure on magnetic resonance imaging in language- and learning-impaired children. *Archives of Neurology and Psychiatry*, 48(5), 539–545. doi: 10.1001/archneur.1991.00530170103028

Kovas, Y., Haworth, C. M., Dale, P. S., & Plomin, R. (2007). The genetic and environmental origins of learning abilities and disabilities in the early school years. *Monograph of the Society for Research in Child Development*, 72(3), 1–144.

Krain, A. L., & Castellanos, F. X. (2006). Brain development and ADHD. *Clin Psychol Rev*, 26(4), 433–444. doi: 10.1016/j.cpr.2006.01.005

Landerl, K., & Moll, K. (2010). Comorbidity of learning disorders: prevalence and familial transmission. *J Child Psychol Psychiatry*, 51(3), 287–294. doi: 10.1111/j.1469–7610.2009.02164.x

Makris, N., Seidman, L. J., Valera, E. M., Biederman, J., Monuteaux, M. C., Kennedy, D. N., Caviness, V. S., Jr., Bush, G., Crum, K., Brown, A. B., & Faraone, S. V. (2010). Anterior cingulate volumetric alterations in treatment-naive adults with ADHD: a pilot study. *J Atten Disord*, 13(4), 407–413. doi: 10.1177/1087054709351671

Proal, E., Reiss, P. T., Klein, R. G., Mannuzza, S, Gotimer, K, Ramos-Olazagasti, M. A., ... Castellanos, F. X. (2011). Brain gray matter deficits at 33-year follow-up in adults with attention-deficit/hyperactivity disorder established in childhood. *Archives of General Psychiatry*, 68(11), 1122–1134. doi: 10.1001/archgenpsychiatry.2011.117

Reeve, R. (in press). Math Learning Difficulties in Australia. In A. Fritz-Stratmann, V. Haase, & P. Räsänen (Eds), *International Handbook of Math Learning Difficulties: From the Lab to the Classroom*. Sao Paulo, Brazil: Springer.

Silani, G., Frith, U., Demonet, J. F., Fazio, F., Perani, D., Price, C., Frith, C. D., & Paulesu, E. (2005). Brain abnormalities underlying altered activation in dyslexia: a voxel based morphometry study. *Brain*, 128(10), 2453–2461. doi: 10.1093/brain/awh579

Snowling, M. J. (2000). *Dyslexia*. Oxford: Blackwell.

Soriano-Mas, C., Pujol, J., Ortiz, H., Deus, J., Lopez-Sala, A., & Sans, A. (2009). Age-related brain structural alterations in children with specific language impairment. *Hum Brain Mapp*, 30(5), 1626–1636. doi: 10.1002/hbm.20620

Yudin, M. K. (2015). [Specific learning disabilities]. Washington DC: United States Department of Education. Retrieved from www2.ed.gov/policy/speced/guid/idea/memosdcltrs/guidance-on-dyslexia-10–2015.pdf

10

Intervention for dyscalculic learners

LEVEL OF EXPLANATION	MEASURES	EDUCATIONAL CONTEXT
BEHAVIOURAL	Number sense Chapter 2	Society, school and home Chapter 8
COGNITIVE	Starter kit for learning arithmetic Chapter 3 Core deficit as the cause of dyscalculia Chapter 4	Assessment Chapter 9
	Development of arithmetic Chapter 5	**Intervention Chapter 10**
NEURAL	Brain structures and functions Chapter 6	Policy Chapter 11
	GENETIC AND OTHER CAUSES Chapter 7	

The approach to intervention advocated in this book is based on three foundations. First, my experience of working with an outstanding specialist teacher of dyscalculics, the late Dorian Yeo. She co-founded Emerson House, a specialist teaching facility for children with dyscalculia, dyslexia and other developmental disorders. Her methods were both innovative and influential. Many, perhaps most, of the best teachers of dyscalculic learners in the UK have been taught by her, or follow her methods. Alas, there are still all too few specialist teachers (see Chapter 11 on policy). Although Dorian and I came to dyscalculia from completely different directions, we agreed that a domain-specific core capacity underpins number concepts and arithmetic, and that this is based on sets and operations on sets. We also took the view that it was a deficit in this core capacity that caused dyscalculia. Therefore, teaching dyscalculics should be based on teaching sets and the relationships within and between the sets, before going on to work with symbolic calculation. This prescription will come as no surprise to primary school teachers.

Her second principle was that teaching must be based on careful diagnostic assessment and activities should *adapt* to each individual learner's current state of understanding. In the case of dyscalculia, understanding on Monday may be lost by Tuesday and will need refreshing. Much of what I will say in this chapter is based on our book, *Dyscalculia Guidance* (Butterworth & Yeo, 2004). It provides a systematic sequence of activities that progresses from sets to abstract representations of number, and a good teacher will adapt the ordering of this sequence to the individual learner.

Among those who learned from Dorian, were Jane Emerson and Patricia Babtie, who went on to write four books (so far) on dyscalculia. Their books *The Dyscalculia Assessment* and *The Dyscalculia Solution* (Emerson & Babtie, 2013; 2014) were specifically designed to make Dorian's approach accessible to the non-specialist. They give detailed information on how to assess strengths and weaknesses in arithmetic and propose activities that can help the learner rehearse and extend areas of strength, and strengthen areas of weakness.

Second, our book said nothing about how digital technologies could provide *adaptive* activities tailored to the learner's current level of competence. In the ideal case, these activities will be *digital Dorian* – progression from sets to calculations with numerals. Here I have depended critically on the work of Diana Laurillard, Professor of Learning with Digital Technologies, at the UCL Institute of Education. We have collaborated to develop digital games for dyscalculics and early learners based on relevant actions, maximally informative feedback and adaptation to the learner's current level of competence. One important aspect of digital games is that other people – teachers, parents, students – don't see you fail. We think this alone can reduce fear.

The third foundation is what we have discovered recently about the neural system for basic numerical processes, described in Chapter 6, and also about how the brain learns. In simple terms, the brain learns by a prediction-error process (see Frith, 2007 for a clear non-technical account of this idea). The brain predicts the result of an action, and in the light of feedback may modify its prediction to attain or get closer to the target. Think of an archer aiming at a target. The archer predicts that the current action will hit the bullseye. Let's say that in fact the arrow flies to the left of the bull. Given this information, next time the archer will predict that aiming a bit more to the right will minimize the error and designs the new action in light of that prediction. Now, if the feedback is simply whether the arrow did or did not hit the bullseye, the archer will not have enough information to make an appropriate modification, and this could lead to a bigger error, for example, if the new prediction results in aiming a bit more to the left.

The other important point of this example, is that the action, aiming the arrow, is relevant to attaining the goal – hitting the bullseye. This is quite different from selecting one response from several options, as in a multiple-choice questionnaires. Selecting one from a set of alternatives is too general a type of response: it applies as much to selecting the capital of Mali from a set of alternatives, as selecting the correct solution for 4 + 5 =? From 7, 8 or 9. What's more, this kind of activity allows guessing, and indeed with time pressure, may encourage guessing. This has two main undesirable properties: first, you can respond without thinking about the content of the question, and, second, if you pick the wrong alternative you don't know why you were wrong: there is not enough information in the feedback.

The aim of this chapter is to outline the main principles that should govern an intervention programme, rather than provide a detailed teaching scheme. In any case, these are already available in the books I mentioned above.

Principles of dyscalculia intervention

I have argued that dyscalculia can be understood as a deficit in the most basic capacity for number – the "core deficit" – upon which everything in number work is built. What this means in practice is that most of what *you* find blindingly obvious – so obvious, in fact, that you don't even realise that you know it – dyscalculics may struggle with. This is because the relationship between numbers and sets is not secure. Here are some things that you know that dyscalculics may not know (to repeat what I wrote in Chapter 4):

■ Numbers are composed of other numbers: 4 can be composed of 1, 1, 1 and 1, or 2 and 2, etc. The parts of 4 are called "partitions" and there are 5 partitions of 4. These are very easy to see in terms of sets. □□□□ can be broken down into ones (□,□,□,□) into two subsets of two (□□, □□), etc.

■ Addition is commutative: 3 + 5 is the same as 5 + 3
□□□□+□□□□□□ □□□□□□+□□□□

■ Addition and subtraction are inverse operations: if 5 + 3 = 8, then 8 − 5 = 3 and 8 − 3 = 5
(□□□□□) (□□□)

So, if you count the union of the two sets, you get 8, if you take away the set of five it leaves 3, and if you take away the set of three it leaves 5.

It doesn't help that the words used in number work are so ambiguous. Just take the word "five". This could mean a set of five objects, in which case, it would imply all the partitions of five such that the set contains the smaller subsets of four, three, two and one objects. It could mean a rank or a position in an ordering – as in a page number or house number, in which case page five is not bigger than page four, and house five is not bigger than house four, and certainly doesn't contain it. "Five" could also have a non-numerical meaning: Channel 5 on a TV, or on a football shirt. But it is only the set-based meaning – the numerosity of the set – that is relevant to ordinary arithmetic.

Of course, there are problems with the words we use for arithmetical operations. Addition of two numbers is described in many ways, with the operation and its syntactic relations to the addends being quite different. Consider how we might talk about 5 + 3 = 8:

> five and three make eight
> five plus three make eight
> five and three equals eight
> five plus three equals eight
> five plus three is eight
> five add three is/makes/equals eight
> five added to three makes/equals/is eight
> etc.

Subtraction suffers similar, if not worse, language problems:

> Five minus three is/makes/equals two
> Five take away three is/makes/equals two
> Three from five is/makes/equals two
> Five less three is/makes/equals two
> etc.

If the learner is already struggling to understand the meaning of the numbers and the meaning of operations on the numbers, these different ways of talking about the same arithmetical operation can only be confusing. Dorian and I recommend that

> Teachers should be prepared to re-phrase what they say until they are sure that pupils have understood what they mean. Pupils should also be encouraged to describe concepts and procedures in simple terms and to translate mathematical symbols into language that makes sense to them.

In fact, in *Dyscalculia Guidance*, we carefully note likely problems with language and what to do about them.

So, to help dyscalculics begin making progress, intervention has to start by exercises to strengthen the basic capacity to represent numerosities as sets and to link them to number words and numerals.

Dorian and I argued, that:

- Intervention is based on understanding basic number concepts.
- The sequence of activities is carefully structured to adapt to the learner's current level of understanding.
- It should make arithmetic learning a positive experience.

So-called traditional learning, or learning important aspects of number work by rote, through repetitive drill, does not help dyscalculic learners. Classroom studies show that dyscalculics do not remember rote learned facts or procedures.

If dyscalculics – and other learners whatever their age – are to remember numbers and their relationships, they have to be able to *make sense of numbers.*

Making sense of numbers

A reasonable understanding of number concepts, number structures and calculation procedures helps support dyscalculics in the difficult process of trying to learn and remember them. This means that intervention has to begin with activities designed to strengthen number sense.

Concrete materials

As I have argued in earlier chapters, numbers are abstract: they are abstract properties of sets, and sets themselves are abstract. However, members of sets can be concrete objects. We have found that dyscalculics are able to make much better sense of number work when the teachers use *concrete materials* to *illustrate* sets, such as beads, counters, blocks or toys.

Composing and decomposing sets of blocks, accompanied by counting, help dyscalculic learners understand the foundational concept that numbers are made out of other numbers. This is so obvious to most people, that it may seem odd that teaching should stress this, but dyscalculics may not have already grasped this. Counting helps the learner reflect on the critical relationship between number symbols – words and numerals – and their basis in sets. It is important therefore to organise the objects into patterns or structures that give meaning to the symbols. Because our system of number symbols is based on ten, ten-based materials such as Dienes Blocks, Cuisenaire Rods and tens-structured number tracks or tens-structured beads, will help the learner understand the meaning of the symbols.

Typical early learners can make generalisations from what they already know. For example, a typical early learner can reason from knowing that 2 + 2 makes 4, to derived facts such as 2 + 3 makes 5. Not all dyscalculics can do this, but from working with sets of concrete materials can promote this kind of generalisation: that is, putting two blocks together with counting out another two blocks plus another block to make three, can help the child make and understand this generalisation

Adapt teaching to the current level of understanding

Typical numeracy lessons cover number work too rapidly for dyscalculic learners, and they frequently become confused if work proceeds too quickly.

It is not sufficient that the teaching should be slower, it must be *adaptive* to the learner's current level of understanding. That is, in Vygotsky's terms, "the distance between the actual developmental level as determined by independent problem solving and the level of potential development as determined through problem solving under adult guidance, or in collaboration with more capable peers" (Vygotsky, 1978, p. 86). This has come to be known as "the zone of prox-imal development".

Even work that seemed to have made sense in the last lesson, may be forgotten at the next lesson. This means that teaching should proceed in very small, pro-gressive steps, and teachers also need to provide dyscalculic learners with exten-sive practice. As Dorian and I wrote,

> From the outset, dyscalculics need to acquire … the foundation understandings that they fail to internalise. To help dyscalculics *retain* these key understandings and continue making progress, teachers have to find ways of continuing to put these foundation understandings in place for as long as pupils need to be reminded of them.
>
> (Butterworth & Yeo, 2004, 9)

In our study of one intervention programme – "Numbers Count" - that is gen-erally effective for low attaining five and six-year-olds (Dowrick, 2015), we found that it didn't help those assessed as dyscalculic (Iuculano et al., in preparation). Now Numbers Count was not designed with dyscalculic learners in mind, and it may be that with more practice it may have been more effective (I discuss how digital technology can provide more practice below).

Carefully limit all memory demands

Teachers have to limit the *long-term memory* demands made on dyscalculic pupils. This implies reducing the number of facts to be learned, and helping the learner reason from an understanding of the basic concepts and arithmetical principles. Let me give a simple example. It is very important that the leaner knows the number bonds to ten, that is, the combinations of numbers that add up to ten. Now, the teacher *could* teach that 3 + 7 makes 10, and, separately, that 7 + 3 makes 10, and drill each fact by rote until both can be retrieved from memory with some fluency. However, it would be better for the child to understand that 3 + 7 and 7 + 3 are equivalent by, for example, using two sets of seven objects and three objects and demonstrating the equivalence of the union operations on the sets: bringing the three to the seven, or the seven to the three, and then counting the union. In this way, not only is long-term memory load reduced – only one fact to remember – but the learner will have an understanding of the commutativity of addition based on operations on sets.

Teachers should limit the *Working Memory* demands so that learners can focus on understanding the basic concepts and principles. As we will see below, anx-iety can reduce working memory capacity, and this in turn can affect how well the task is carried out, especially when the task is complex. What's more, com-plex arithmetical tasks which make heavy demands on Working Memory may in themselves induce anxiety, which in turn, reduces Working Memory capacity, which in turn impairs performance, which in turn can induce anxiety, and so on.

To go back to the example of understanding the principles of addition: limiting Working Memory demands implies, and this again will come as no surprise to reflective teachers, starting with simple additions

Provide an intensive, cyclical teaching programme

Teachers should provide sufficient repetition or practice of material and find ways to "put back" any knowledge which has been forgotten, and this means adapting practice to individual differences in motivation as well as level of understanding.

Some dyscalculic learners respond to variety, and prefer teachers to change learning materials or practice activities quite regularly, while other dyscalculic learners prefer familiar materials, familiar activities and familiar exercises.

It should be clear to the learner that practice activities and games are not tests, but are designed to help the learner learn.

Guide pupils carefully from concrete work to abstract work

Dorian and I took the view that "Most maths teaching becomes too abstract too quickly", and this is particularly true of dyscalculic learners. On the other hand, it is not helpful if dyscalculic learners *remain* dependent on concrete tools, and this means designing a programme for the transition from concrete to abstract. This means progressively linking representations of sets to number words (one, two, three ...), to number symbols (1, 2, 3 ...) and representations of operations on sets to the words for arithmetical operations (add, take away, makes, equals...) and the symbols (+, -, = ...).

So, we developed methods for managing the transition from concrete (visual) representations of numerosity to numbers. For example, teachers can link sets of dots or other objects to numbers using "triads" to depict partitions, as in Figure 10.1.

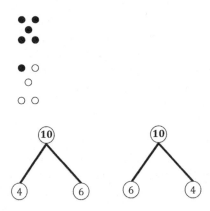

Figure 10.1 Two ways of representing partitions of 10.

This makes it easy to understand the partitions of 10 in terms of sets, in term of numbers, and in terms of their relationships.

Here are the stages from concrete to abstract that Dorian and I set out in our book, and subsequently developed by her colleagues, Jane Emerson and Patricia Babtie:

- In the early stages of learning any aspect of numbers, teachers guide pupils to reason using concrete materials, for example, by splitting and combining sets of objects.
- In an intermediate stage, pupils may start out by building a model or by using concrete materials. The model or materials are then covered and pupils are encouraged to think through problems related to the concrete work. Pupils may use the materials to check their solutions or if they become "stuck". Alternatively, teachers may leave a familiar material in view. Dyscalculic pupils are encouraged to figure out solutions mentally, but they have the reassuring knowledge that they can use the concrete materials to confirm their solutions or to remind them of "how they could think". Some learners need a *diagrammatic stage* drawing diagrams of the concrete materials. Babtie writes,

  > Many people I have taught are not able to "think through problems related to the concrete work" because they have not been able to internalize the image/concept from the concrete. Sometimes it takes extensive tuition at this level. What is often clear to me is that the pupil may not "see" what I see when we are both looking at the same object. Only by learning to draw do they start to elicit the relevant information and only then can they think about it.

  > (Personal communication)

- Finally, abstract spoken or written questions are given to dyscalculic pupils to solve. At first, teachers may start out by making a link to concrete work: teachers may directly ask pupils to picture a specific model to help them to figure out a solution. In time, dyscalculic pupils are given "bare" number problems to solve. In all abstract work, teachers should make clear that concrete materials would always be made available, should they be needed.

Digital interventions

Dorian's activities for dyscalculic learners are designed to discourage guessing – often the first response of the dyscalculic – and to maximize the information provided in the feedback: is the result too big, or too small, not just right or wrong. Guessing in a task that just offers a choice of alternatives, can associate the wrong answer with question. So, if dyscalculic Johnny selects 28 as half of 72, this may stick in his mind even if he is told that this wrong, and is subsequently told that it is 36. Modelling brain function suggests that the brain adds the new information to existing information, but does not "overwrite" the old information. This principle should be built in to any digital activity.

Digital activities can be, should be and must be *adaptive*. The thousands of digital maths games on the internet typically select the next task at random, whereas what they should do, and could do, is make them adaptive. That is, they could use the data from the learner's performance to determine what the next task should be. Of course, this is not a trivial matter. It could take accuracy or fluency, or both, into account in determining the next task. Here a computer has an advantage over the teacher: it does not forget, whereas even the best teacher, perhaps with many pupils, may forget what Johnny did last week. The computer, by contrast, will store in its memory exactly what Johnny did yesterday or last week, to decide what Johnny should do today. Now, if Johnny has forgotten what he learned last time he did the activity, a suitable adaptive algorithm could select an earlier and easier task for Johnny to try next, just like a good and sensitive teacher would do.

The aim of digital interventions, as with teacher interventions, is to make numbers meaningful for the learner, and it should follow the same principles. I give an example from our digital game NumberBeads.

Start with virtual concrete materials representing sets:

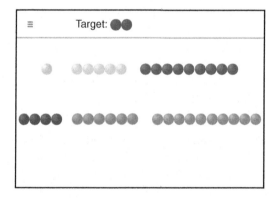

Figure 10.2 Level 1 in NumberBeads. Here the learner tries to make the target by splitting sets and/or combining sets using two simple "mechanics": drawing a line to split a set, or moving one set to combine with another.

Adapt teaching to the current level of understanding.

Practicing splitting and combining sets to make a target helps the learner understand the set basis of arithmetic: combining sets is the basis of addition, splitting a set into subsets in the basis of subtraction. As the learner progresses, the game adapts to increase the size of the targets. To support this stage of understanding, the set size is always the same colour: two is always red, four is always purple, and so on.

The game progresses to the next level where the sets are linked to digits.

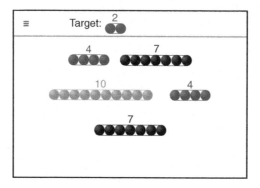

Figure 10.3 Level 2 in NumberBeads where the sets of virtual concrete objects are linked to digits.

Level 2 provides the learner with the opportunity to make the cognitive link between a set of particular size and the digit representing that size. Again, the game adapts to learner understanding by progressively increasing the size of the target.

Progress in small steps

In Level 3, the colours are removed so that the learner has to focus on the number of beads in the sets, which encourages counting them and learning to make the cognitive link between sets, digits and counting words.

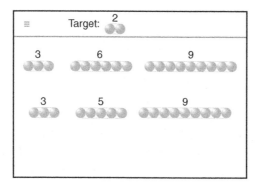

Figure 10.4 Level 3 in NumberBeads.

Make the transition to numerals unsupported by sets

In Level 4, manipulations of digits are animated to reveal the underlying sets: so, bringing 3 and 2 together reveal the set of three in green, the set of two in red, and the resultant set of five in yellow. In Level 5, the learner is operating just with the digits.

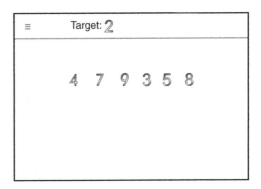

Figure 10.5 Levels 4 and 5 in NumberBeads. Here a digit can be partitioned by clicking on it. For example, clicking on the 4 could yield 2 and 2, or 3 and 1. Numbers can be combined by placing them adjacently.

Neural basis of learning

In Chapter 6, I described the arithmetical network in the brain that connects the left frontal lobe with the left and right parietal lobes. In general terms, we know that the structure of brain regions and their connections change in response to experiences, including learning. When a new fact is learned, for example *that 36 is half of 72*, this does not mean that a previous guess, for example that it is 28, will be overwritten. Rather, the associations among half, 36 and 72 will be strengthened and those among half, 28 and 72 will be weakened. However, the erroneous links will still be in the brain. This is an argument for abandoning multiple choice questionnaires (MCQs) as a response mode in intervention, because MCQs encourage guessing, which in turn create erroneous links in the brain (Zorzi et al., 2005).

It is now also believed that the internal structure of the neurons themselves are modified by learning (Gallistel, 2017).

The general principles of how the brain learns are clear, though the precise mechanisms in particular learning situations can be complex. Typically, the brain starts with expectations based on prior experience. These could be of what will happen next, or what will be the effect of an action. The expectation can be in the form of precise predictions, as in the case of the archer (above). Learning involves using informative feedback to minimize the difference between the predictions based on prior experience and the outcome. In this way, the basis for future predictions is updated. Next time should therefore be better. Learning new concepts or adding new facts to memory is more abstract that aiming an arrow at a target, but the principles will be the same.

In everyday life, predictions are deployed to construct an action to obtain a reward or to avoid distress or loss. There have been many studies exploring how the value attributed to the reward or the loss affects the prediction, and how the reward networks are involved (Frith, 2007).

Unfortunately, there has been very little research on how the brain learns mathematics specifically. One thing that has been discovered is that learning new facts or practicing new strategies reduces the mental load required for prediction, planning an action and checking the outcome, and therefore reduces activation in the brain area where these processes are carried out, the frontal lobes (Ischebeck et al., 2007; Ischebeck et al., 2006; Zhao et al., 2017).

There is even less research on the effects of learning on the dyscalculic brain. One study examined the brain changes in seven to nine-year-olds induced by a systematic eight week intervention on children with "moderate to severe mathematical learning disabilities" (MLD) (Iuculano et al., 2015). The intervention included several aspects of symbolic arithmetic (e.g. 3 + 4 = 7), without an explicit focus on the relationship between symbols and sets. The intervention was designed to improve calculation efficiency and, to a lesser extent, promote understanding of arithmetical concepts and principles:

- speeded retrieval of arithmetical facts
- relations within and between addition and subtraction
- counting on and retrieval processes

One very striking finding was that this intervention reduced overall activation in the arithmetic fronto-parietal network. This is in line with many studies showing that practice reduces cognitive load and hence the amount of brain activation needed to carry out a task successfully. Before intervention, the patterns of brain activity were very different in the MLD learners compared with the typical learners. After intervention, the patterns of activity were indistinguishable. The MLD children were classified by using standardized tests of arithmetic – Numerical Operations and Mathematical Reasoning from WIAT II (Wechsler, 2002), but there was no test of their ability to enumerate or compare sets of objects. This means that, at least according to the position taken in this book, that we cannot tell which of these children had a "core deficit" based on their performance on the enumeration or comparison of sets of objects.

Fear

My colleague, Patricia Babtie, has written, "The biggest obstacle to learning is fear" (Babtie, 2017, p. xii), and there has been much research into the effects "maths anxiety". Indeed, Anna Bevan and I have recorded the nature and the effects of anxiety in 15 focus groups of nine-year-olds, three in five schools in London. Each group comprised learners of similar mathematical competence – low, medium and high. We recorded each group, and transcribed what was said verbatim (Bevan & Butterworth, 2007).

Here you can see that the low ability children reported low self-esteem, feeling stupid, and frustrated.

School 1 (low ability group)

> Child 5: It makes me feel left out, sometimes.
> Child 2: Yeah.
> Child 5: When I like – when I don't know something, I wish that I was like a clever person and I blame it on myself –
> Child 4: I would cry and I wish I was at home with my mum and it would be - I won't have to do any maths –

School 2 (low ability group)

> Moderator: How does it make people feel in a maths lesson when they lose track?
> Child 1: Horrible.
> Moderator: Horrible? … Why's that?
> Child 1: I don't know.
> Child 3 (whispers): He does know.
> Moderator: Just a guess.
> Child 1: You feel stupid.

School 3 (low ability group)

> Child 5: I feel like screaming and saying "why are you doing this, why are you doing this?" and I feel like punching the teachers!

Of course, even at the age of nine, children are well aware that maths is important for their futures, and they are concerned that they are not learning maths as well as their classmates.

School 3 (low ability group)

> Child 1: You might forget what the teacher has taught you –
> Child 3: All you can be is a dustbin man.

School 5 (low ability group)

> Child 2: If you don't learn, yeah, you won't have a good job and you'll be a dustbin man.

There is extensive evidence that anxiety can reduce Working Memory capacity (e.g. Eysenck & Calvo, 1992), and this in turn can affect mathematical performance especially on tasks with high Working Memory load (Ashcraft & Krause, 2007) (see Chapter 5 for more on the role of Working Memory capacity and mathematics performance); however, there is a difference between poor performance and dyscalculia. Anxiety is usually assessed by questionnaire (Faust et al., 1996; Richardson & Suinn, 1972; Wu et al., 2012; Wu & Menon, 2012).

Here is an example of a recent questionnaire called the *Scale for Early Mathematics Anxiety (SEMA)* used to assess maths anxiety when carrying out a mathematics task and when in a maths class.

> Instructions: "Now I'm going to show you some math questions. I want you to read each question and pretend that you are going to answer it. Then I want you to tell me how nervous answering that question makes you feel. So remember, you do not actually have to answer the questions, but I just want you to pretend you are going to answer them and see how it makes you feel. It could make you feel not nervous AT ALL, a little nervous, somewhat nervous, very nervous, or VERY, VERY nervous.
>
> 1. George bought two pizzas that had six slices each. How many total slices did George have to share with his friends?
> 2. Is this right? 9 + 7 = 18.
> 3. How much money does Annie have if she has two dimes and four pennies?

There are ten questions like this and then ten when you have to pretend that you are in a maths class.

Clearly, there will be individual differences in how well children of seven to nine years can answer these questions, including how well children are at recognizing and remembering their mental states. Nevertheless, there was a significant relationship between SEMA scores and a standardized maths test (WIAT-II (Wechsler, 2002)). What score on the SEMA counts as maths anxious? One rigorous recent study sets the bar as the 10% most anxious (Devine et al., 2017), but other studies use other cut-offs. This study also showed that 77% of children with high anxiety had typical or high mathematics performance. On the other hand, children with dyscalculia (here 6% of the sample) were twice as likely to have high anxiety.

Of course, it is important to distinguish between what psychologists call "trait anxiety", that is, whether the learner is generally anxious, and "state anxiety", where the learner is made anxious by maths. Trait anxiety does not seem to be related to maths performance, while state anxiety – maths anxiety – is related (Wu et al., 2012). Anxious learners not only become anxious or fearful when carrying out maths tasks, they will also *worry* about how they will perform. Worrying itself creates problems. If learners are worrying about how they will perform at the same time as they are carrying out the maths task, this will reduce the available working memory capacity that can be devoted to carrying it out (see Trezise & Reeve (2016) for a study of worry in older learners).

Now correlation is not cause, as we all know. Are learners anxious simply because they are not very good at maths and get anxious about any task they are not good at? Or, are they anxious about maths and this causes poorer performance? Or perhaps both. Maths anxiety is present in younger children, as we have seen, but it seems to be worse in older learners (Dowker, 2005), which suggests that maths anxiety can build up with repeated exposure. If anxiety leads to avoidance and avoidance leads to falling further behind one's classmates, this would give rise to a vicious circle in which both anxiety is likely to increase and age-related performance to decline still further. Indeed, in our interviews with teachers, this was their impression too. As one said to us:

> Teacher MM: The gap will get bigger and bigger unless they give them a chance to catch up…. So I think for them, I would prefer them not to have the Numeracy Hour, but just to focus on those basic skills.

So why are individuals maths anxious? This seems to be a rarely asked question. We have seen from our focus group study, that low ability learners are unhappy in the numeracy lesson. Part of the reason seems to be that they are unable to understand the lesson content.

School 4 (low ability group)

> Child 2: I sometimes don't understand whatever she (the teacher) says.

School 2 (low ability group)

> Child 2: I don't forget it, I don't even know what she's saying.

School 4 (low ability group)

> Child 5: Oh, there's this really hard thing, about when you're doing times – Miss S_____ says you can't take away this number, but I keep on taking away, I don't understand one single bit of it.
> Child 3: You've got to times it, not take it away!
> Child 2: Yeah, I agree with you.

School 2 (low ability group)

> Child 3: When you listen to the teacher, then you turn your head and you don't know nothing…. If I remember something, and then the teacher says "stop for a second, just listen to me" then as soon as she talks, yeah, and we come back, we do work, and I say "what do I have to do?" I always forget.

But there is more to it than failing to understand the content. As one teacher put it to us: "Some of them have got an emotional thing about it, just – they're just scared of maths". Babtie puts it like this: "Repeated failure and *humiliation* quickly turns to anxiety and fear" (Babtie, 2017, p. xii, my italics).

Let us pick up on the idea of humiliation. In class, everyone can see you fail. In our focus group study, it was clear that other children were well aware of the children who were failing.

School 3 (high ability group)

> Child 1: She's like – she's like all upset and miserable, and she don't like being teased.
> Child 4: Yeah, and then she goes hide in the corner – nobody knows where she is and she's crying there.

School 4 (high ability group)

> Child 5: They sometimes - sometimes you can see them cry.

School 5 (high ability group)

> Child 5: Yeah, and then they waste their time crying.

What is more those who are failing are well aware of the responses from their more able peers. Here's what one child said:

> Child 3: He just comes up to us and says "ha ha – you don't know anything – you are so dumb" and then he asks me, like, questions like "thousand times thousand" which he knows and I don't know.

School 1 (high ability group)

> Child 3: And sometimes what happens is Miss J gives us partners –
> Child 5: Which is the worst.
> Child 3: And you get really exasperated, because, you know, they might not know the answer, and you think "oh, come on! You know the answer!"
> Child 5: You usually get someone who's not so clever.

School 5 (high ability group)

> Child 3: Some people – some people, the teacher asks "anybody who doesn't understand?" And they don't put their hand up, because they think that – they're – they're too shy.
> Child 2: They're too frightened, that someone will tease them.

Teachers

Anna Bevan also interviewed the teachers of these learners. Teachers generally recognised the emotional problems attendant on constant failure in class:

> Teacher LS: I think they tend to get very frustrated, if they can't understand anything.
> Teacher SW: … some of them have got an emotional thing about it, just – they're just scared of maths.

Teacher AS: He doesn't have any self-confidence in asking, and he's – and it all compounds itself, you know, one difficulty leads to the other.

The teachers told us about the consequences of a learner's failure to understand:

Teacher CP: I think a child who's struggling is either likely to be disruptive or to be – or to opt out.

Teacher JL: … lots of times they're trying to cover it up. And sometimes they'll cover it up – they'd rather be told off for being naughty than being told off that they're thick.

There were emotional consequences for the teachers too.

Teacher ML1: I really feel very guilty that I'm not giving them the attention they need.

Teacher VW: If I could just focus on them [the strugglers] that would be fine. And if I could focus on the others that would be fine as well, but trying to split – be split between the two is quite hard really.

Humiliation can happen whenever there is an opportunity for the learner to be judged, and judged adversely. This means in every maths lessons – five times a week in most schools – there is a risk of teasing and disparagement from other learners but also from the teacher. The teacher may not mean to humiliate the learner, but even saying something like "You ought to know that," can be distressing.

At home, similarly, parents can think that the child who is doing badly is not trying hard enough because they are failing tests. If it's maths competence, often a proxy for intelligence, parents can think their child is just not very bright. All this can have an effect on self-confidence, self-esteem, self-efficacy, or on happiness and misery.

There is also vicious circle of performance well below the current target, which is usually set by others, such as teachers or parents, leading to anxiety, avoidance, falling even farther behind, leading to more anxiety and avoidance and so on. Anna Bevan and I created Figure 10.6 to illustrate the process.

Breaking the circle

Anna and I proposed the following scheme to help the anxious child, and especially the fearful dyscalculic:

1. The vicious circle can be broken by interventions targeted at each child's current level of understanding. Structured teaching, small steps, use of concrete materials, slow pace, transparent language and plenty encouragement are essential to effective intervention. This will lead to happier experiences of doing maths.
2. Adaptive digital games can be helpful, since they are self-paced, structured and private.

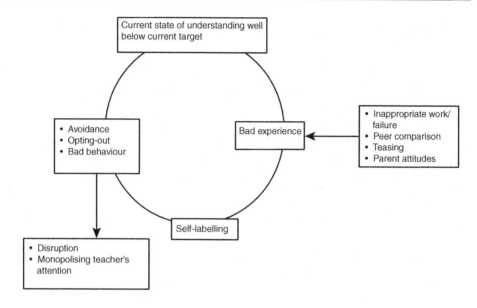

Figure 10.6 The anxiety vicious circle.

3. Drills – rote learning of materials that are not understood – are not useful and can be counterproductive because they induce stress without helping the child understand the concepts.

4. Low ability children should be screened from the scrutiny of their peers to prevent teasing and stigmatisation of their failures.

5. For dyscalculics, improving understanding will be slow, and needs to proceed at a different pace from the rest of the class.

Summary

■ Because dyscalculics have a core deficit, interventions should start by focusing on sets and operations on sets that underlie arithmetic.

■ The content of the lessons should be systematically structured so that the learner can progress from concrete representations of sets to drawing diagrammatic representations and then to the familiar symbols of numbers and arithmetical operations.

■ Interventions should adapt systematically to the learner's current level of competence and understanding.

■ Initially dyscalculics will have difficulty remembering what they have learned, and will need reminding.

■ The pedagogical method, whether with the teacher or with digital support, should require the learner to predict the outcome of a relevant action and provide maximally informative feedback about the result of the action, and enable the learner to correct an incorrect action.

■ Interventions should be enjoyable for the learner and not stressful.

References

Ashcraft, M. H., & Krause, J. A. (207). Working memory, math performance, and math anxiety. *Psychonomic Bulletin & Review*, 14, 243–248. doi: 10.3758/BF03194059

Babtie, P. (2017). *100 Ideas for Primary Teachers: Numeracy Difficulties and Dyscalculia*. London: Bloomsbury Education.

Bevan, A., & Butterworth, B. (2007). The responses to maths disabilities in the classroom. Draft 2002. Retrieved from www.mathematicalbrain.com/pdf/2002BEVANBB.PDF

Butterworth, B., & Yeo, D. (2004). *Dyscalculia Guidance: Helping Pupils with Specific Learning Difficulties in Maths*. London: David Fulton.

Devine, A., Hill, F., Carey, E., & Szűcs, D. (2017). Cognitive and Emotional Math Problems Largely Dissociate: Prevalence of Developmental Dyscalculia and Mathematics Anxiety. *Journal of Educational Psychology* (Advance online publication.). doi: 10.1037/edu0000222

Dowker, A. D. (2005). *Individual Differences in Arithmetic: Implications for Psychology, Neuroscience and Education*. Hove, East Sussex: Psychology Press.

Dowrick, N. (2015). Numbers count: a large-scale intervention for young children who struggle with mathematics. In R. Cohen Kadosh & A. Dowker (Eds), *Oxford Handbook of Numerical Cognition* (pp. 1099–1117). Oxford: OUP.

Emerson, J., & Babtie, P. (2013). *The Dyscalculia Assessment* (Second edition). London: Bloomsbury Education.

Emerson, J., & Babtie, P. (2014). *The Dyscalculia Solution: Teaching Number Sense*. London: Bloomsbury Education.

Eysenck, M. W., & Calvo, M. G. (1992). Anxiety and performance – the processing efficiency theory. *Cognition & Emotion*, 6(6), 409–434.

Faust, M. W., Ashcraft, M. H., & Fleck, D. E. (1996). Mathematics anxiety effects in simple and complex addition. *Mathematical Cognition*, 2(1), 25–62.

Frith, C. D. (2007). *Making up the Mind: How the Brain Creates our Mental World*. Oxford: Blackwell Publishing.

Gallistel, C. R. (2017). The Coding Question. *Trends in Cognitive Sciences*, 21(7), 498–508. doi: 10.1016/j.tics.2017.04.012

Ischebeck, A., Zamarian, L., Egger, Karl, Schocke, M., & Delazer, M. (2007). Imaging early practice effects in arithmetic. *NeuroImage*, 36(3), 993–1003. doi: 10.1016/j.neuroimage.2007.03.051

Ischebeck, A., Zamarian, L., Siedentopf, C., Koppelstatter, F., Benke, T., Felber, S., & Delazer, M. (2006). How specifically do we learn? Imaging the learning of multiplication and subtraction. *NeuroImage*, 30(4), 1365–1375.

Iuculano, T., Dowrick, N., & Butterworth, B. (in preparation). The Effectiveness of the "Numbers Count" Intervention for Learners with Dyscalculia.

Iuculano, T., Rosenberg-Lee, Miriam, Richardson, Jennifer, Tenison, Caitlin, Fuchs, Lynn, Supekar, Kaustubh, & Menon, Vinod. (2015). Cognitive tutoring induces widespread neuroplasticity and remediates brain function in children with mathematical learning disabilities. *Nat Commun*, 6. doi: 10.1038/ncomms9453

Richardson, F. C., & Suinn, R. M. (1972). The Mathematics Anxiety Rating Scale. *Journal of Counseling Psychology*, 19, 551–554.

Trezise, Kelly, & Reeve, Robert A. (2016). Worry and working memory influence each other iteratively over time. *Cognition and Emotion*, 30(2), 353–368. doi: 10.1080/0269 9931.2014.1002755

Wechsler, D. (2002). *Wechsler Individual Achievement Test* (2nd edition). San Antonio, TX: The Psychological Corporation.

Wu, S., Amin, Hitha, Barth, Maria, Malcarne, Vanessa, & Menon, Vinod. (2012). Math Anxiety in Second and Third Graders and Its Relation to Mathematics Achievement. *Frontiers in Psychology*, 3(162). doi: 10.3389/fpsyg.2012.00162

Wu, S., & Menon, V. (2012). Scale for Early Mathematics Anxiety (SEMA) in Young Children. Retrieved from www.scsnl.stanford.edu

Zhao, Hui, Li, Xiaoxi, Karolis, V., Feng, Yi, Niu, Haijing, & Butterworth, B. (2018). Arithmetic learning modifies the functional connectivity of the fronto-parietal network. *Cortex*. doi: 10.1016/j.cortex.2018.07.016

Zorzi, M., Stoianov, I., & Umilta, C. (2005). Computational modelling of numerical cognition. In J. I. D. Campbell (Ed.), *Handbook of Mathematical Cognition* (pp. 67–84). Hove: Psychology Press.

Policy

What to do about dyscalculia locally and nationally

LEVEL OF EXPLANATION	MEASURES	EDUCATIONAL CONTEXT
BEHAVIOURAL	Number sense Chapter 2	Society, school and home Chapter 8
COGNITIVE	Starter kit for learning arithmetic Chapter 3 Core deficit as the cause of dyscalculia Chapter 4	Assessment Chapter 9
	Development of arithmetic Chapter 5	Intervention Chapter 10
NEURAL	Brain structures and functions Chapter 6	**Policy Chapter 11**
	GENETIC AND OTHER CAUSES Chapter 7	

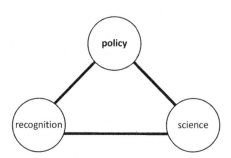

Figure 11.1 The virtuous triangle. When there is improvement in one node, it can, and often will, improve the other nodes. Better policy can promote better science and improve wider recognition. Better recognition can prompt better policy; and better science can lead to better policy and better recognition.

Dyscalculia is not widely recognized in most countries. This means that dyscalculics are neglected, and their life prospects seriously reduced. It does not have to be like this. A few countries recognize the handicap and have laws and policies designed to identify the sufferers and alleviate their suffering.

Policies depend on recognizing that there is a specific problem, and recognition depends on accessible evidence. There could be a policy to identify and explain the problem. This needs science. The science made accessible, can lead to wider recognition, which in turn can inform policy. This is why I stress the virtuous circle: impact at any node can have impact on the other two nodes.

Policy

Educational policy is necessarily political because education is about transmitting and preserving the national culture, which is why governments are interested. Governments introduce changes that it hopes will create a new and different national culture. This may mean trying to erase the legacy of previous governments. Think of Trump's attempts to erase Obama's legacy. What has this got to do with dyscalculia?

The current UK government seeks not only to erase the legacy of the Labour government (1997 to 2010) but even the Coalition government in which it was the senior partner (2010 to 2015). The Labour government had a clear official definition of dyscalculia that is consistent with the one presented in this book:

> Dyscalculia is a condition that affects the ability to acquire arithmetical skills. Dyscalculic learners may have difficulty understanding simple number concepts, lack an intuitive grasp of numbers, and have problems learning number facts and procedures. Even if they produce a correct answer or use a correct method, they may do so mechanically and without confidence..... Purely dyscalculic learners who have difficulties only with number will have cognitive and language abilities in the normal range, and may excel in nonmathematical subjects.

> (DfES, 2001)

In an article in the British newspaper, *The Daily Telegraph*, back in 2002, a DfES spokesman said:

> We provide special educational-needs training for our teachers, and that includes guidelines on dyscalculia. The national numeracy strategy is designed to raise standards in maths for all children and, since September last year, we have been sending out specific information on dyscalculia.

The Coalition government also had a definition in a document that was very hard to locate of its website. In fact, it took a Parliamentary question before

I could locate it. It was in a very useful document called *Advanced Training Materials for Autism; Dyslexia; Speech, Language and Communication; Emotional, Social and Behavioural Difficulties; Moderate Learning Difficulties.* The UK DfE commissioned a linked training resource which was brokered to The Schools, Students and Teachers Network (www.ssatuk.co.uk) and which has been updated by Real Training over the last 18 months and sits on the website www.complexneeds.org. uk. This site provides useful material on the legislative position in the UK on planning educational help mainly for learners with severe, profound or multiple learning difficulties. However, there is nothing on dyscalculia.

There used to be relevant information on the UK government's website, which is now archived and hard to find, indeed almost impossible to find if you don't know that it exists and how to search for it. Figure 11.2 presents a brief and useful guide to arithmetical development, and it mentions but doesn't actually provide a definition of dyscalculia:

> Identifying a specific condition such as dyscalculia can be difficult, given the many explanations for poor performance on maths activities. There are also a wide variety of skills involved in learning mathematics, such as those presented in this mind map.

However, it does reference the DfES document above (though it is not accessible with the link provided). The accompanying material, also no longer accessible, stated

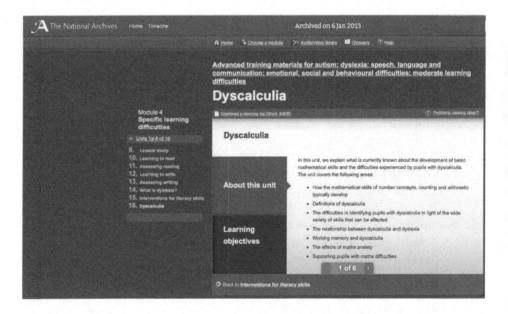

Figure 11.2 The UK Government's mention of dyscalculia in the National Archives.

- Dyscalculics are less accurate and slower at arithmetical operations (Landerl et al., 2004).... Attention should also be paid to how arithmetic problems are solved, and how quickly.
- The defective "number module" hypothesis (Butterworth, 1999) postulates a developing brain has a specialised capacity (number module) for recognising and mentally manipulating numerosities (cardinal values). This is probably hardwired into the brain, and in dyscalculia is thought not to develop normally.

One should also mention that two major policy documents on SEND from the Coalition government have been dropped: the Lamb Inquiry (*Special Educational Needs and Parental Confidence: Report to the Secretary of State on the Lamb Inquiry Review of SEN and Disability Information* (http://dera.ioe.ac.uk/9042/1/Lamb%20 Inquiry%20Review%20of%20SEN%20and%20Disability%20Information.pdf)) and the subsequent policy document, *Support and Aspiration: A New Approach to Special Educational Needs and Disability: Progress and Next Steps,* from the then minister, Sarah Teather. Neither of these explicitly mentioned dyscalculia.

It should be mentioned that these reports nevertheless formed the basis of the Children and Families Act 2014 which reflected the need to strengthen parental voice and choice regarding their child's provision and placement.

As we saw in Chapter 1, dyscalculia policies vary from country to country, and the policies can be incorporated into law. So, for example, the USA has IDEA (the Individuals with Disabilities Education Act), which requires state and local education authorities to carry out appropriate assessments and to provide appropriate help. Italy's Law 170 recognizes dyscalculia as a Specific Learning Disability, and requires appropriate teaching to ensure equal opportunities to develop social and professional capacities, which in turn requires the training of teachers appropriately, wide recognition of the problem, and promotion of early diagnosis and rehabilitation.

By contrast, in the UK there is no such law. That is, there is no legal requirement to assess or to provide support for a dyscalculic person. It may be that, by implication, a dyscalculic is a disabled person. "You're disabled under the Equality Act 2010 if you have a physical or mental impairment that has a 'substantial' and 'long-term' negative effect on your ability to do normal daily activities." (www.gov.uk/definition-of-disability-under-equality-act-2010).

Under the Act, it is against the law to discriminate against someone with a learning disability:

Many people with a learning disability are in work and with the right support can be hard-working and reliable employees.

Adjustments for an employee with a learning disability include:

- altering the recruitment process to allow work trials instead of formal interviews

- using supported employment providers to offer in work support to help learn a role
- providing information in accessible formats

> (www.gov.uk/government/publications/employing-disabled-people-and-people-with-health-conditions/employing-disabled-people-and-people-with-health-conditions)

The webpage then refers us to the British Institute of Learning Disabilities and Mencap, neither of which mentions dyscalculia, or any equivalent term.

There is one specific reference to dyscalculia, and this is to make it clear that a dyscalculic "must not drive" a bus or lorry, but can drive a car though the DVLA (Driver and Vehicle Licensing Authority) must be specifically notified about this. This is not widely known and could be a useful lever to broader recognition of Dyscalculia (www.gov.uk/guidance/psychiatric-disorders-assessing-fitness-to-drive).

There are quasi-governmental bodies that could devise and carry out policy. One is *Every Child Counts*. This is a not-for-profit supported by the DfE that has been running since 2008. This is how it describes its work:

- we create interventions to help children who struggle with reading, writing or numeracy to catch up with their peers, and we train and support teachers and teaching assistants to deliver them.
- we provide professional development to help schools and teachers to raise teaching standards and sustain high achievement for all children.
- we work with many other agencies, academic institutions, charities, mathematics and literacy organisations and specialists on special projects and research. Our aim is to improve learning and teaching for all.

> (https://everychildcounts.edgehill.ac.uk/?s=dyscalculia)

So, what has this to say about dyscalculia? Nothing.

Another potential source of policy ideas about assessment and intervention is *National Numeracy*, a charity, that wants "everyone in the UK to have the numeracy that allows them to make the most of their lives". We have seen in earlier chapters, that dyscalculia can result in people not making the most of their lives – their health, wealth and happiness are made worse.

> Developmental dyscalculia – because of its low profile but high impacts, its priority should be raised. Dyscalculia relates to numeracy and affects between 4–7% of children. It has a much lower profile than dyslexia but can also have substantial impacts: it can reduce lifetime earnings by £114,000 and reduce the probability of achieving five or more GCSEs (A*–C) by 7–20 percentage points. Home and school interventions have again been identified by the Project. Also, technological interventions are extremely

promising, offering individualised instruction and help, although these need more development.

(Beddington et al., 2008)

You might therefore have thought that dyscalculia would be an important part of the work of *National Numeracy*. What does a search for "dyscalculia" on their website come up with? "Top ten dyscalculia reads by Judy Hornigold", that is, her book recommendations as of February 2015. That's it. There is nothing in the work of *National Numeracy* that addresses this important cause of poor numeracy, and, as I have argued in Chapter 10, requires specialized intervention. Notice also the condescending term "reads": not "studies", not "research", not even "books". *National Numeracy* just doesn't take it seriously. One reason may be that they believe that the key to improving numeracy is "a major shift in attitudes". "Negative attitudes are the foremost barrier to making the UK numerate" (www.national numeracy.org.uk/about-us). It would not be surprising that dyscalculics have a negative attitude to numeracy, but this is not why they are dyscalculic.

The UK Office for Standards in Education, Children's Services and Skills (Ofsted), has a document on low numeracy: www.gov.uk/government/uploads/system/uploads/attachment_data/file/417613/Tackling_the_challenge_of_low_numeracy_skills_in_young_people_and_adults.pdf

This contains nothing about dyscalculia.

By contrast, the Irish Department of Education and Skills does. In fact, it lists the Dyscalculia Screener as the test for dyscalculia:

www.education.ie/en/Schools-Colleges/Information/Supports-for-Pupils-with-Special-Needs/List-of-Approved-Assessment-Tests.pdf

So what is to be done to improve policy in a country like the UK, where the education ministry has no policy to provide help for the dyscalculic? Clearly, important players like *National Numeracy* and *Every Child Counts* have not, and presumably will not, make a positive contribution.

Now the UK education ministry is not unique in doing nothing for dyscalculics. Most governments around the world are likely to be in a similar position.

This is where the *Virtuous Triangle* comes in. If these organisations cannot or will not influence government policy, then science and recognition may. The objective, it seems to me, is to ensure that the government, in particular the education ministry, recognises dyscalculia and plans provision for identification and intervention. I'll return to policy below.

Recognition

Without explicit mention by the government, it is not surprising that society at large does not recognize dyscalculia. And without recognition by society (voters), it is not surprising that government does not feel obliged to mention it.

Now dyscalculia is not at the moment as widely recognized as other specific learning difficulties, such as dyslexia, nor other neurodevelopmental disorders such as autism and ADHD. There are UK organizations that are meant to deal with the range of specific learning difficulties such as PATOSS (the Professional Association for teachers and assessors of students with Specific Learning Difficulties) or NASEN (National Association for Special Educational Needs) ignore dyscalculia, but devote considerable resources to dyslexia. Is this because they think that poor literacy is more important than poor numeracy? It's not.

Summarizing a great deal of research, the UK government's then chief scientific adviser wrote, "Developmental dyscalculia is currently the poor relation of dyslexia, with a much lower public profile. But the consequences of dyscalculia are at least as severe as those for dyslexia" (Beddington et al., 2008). This research shows that numeracy difficulties have a bigger effect on life chances than literacy difficulties (Bynner & Parsons, 1997; 2006; Parsons & Bynner, 2005).

Given the importance many governments in the UK and elsewhere have placed on mathematics education, governmental neglect of dyscalculia is perhaps surprising. Here are just a few of the more recent examples of governmental concern with maths education. There was the Cockcroft report in 1982 (Cockcroft, 1982), Adrian Smith's report on post-14 maths (Smith, 2004), and Sir Peter Williams's report on primary maths (Williams, 2008); the US National Research Council's report in 2009 (Cross et al., 2009). The relationship between maths and the economy is well understood by policy makers, and well supported by research. Thus an OECD analysis demonstrated that a nation's standard of maths drives GDP growth (OECD, 2010).

What is less understood is the impact of improving the standard of the lowest performing. If the UK improved the standard of the 11% of children who failed to reach the PISA minimum level (which is not very high), to the minimum level, then the effect on GDP (Gross Domestic Product) growth would be about 0.44% per annum. Not much you might think, but with an average rate of GDP growth of 1.5%, this would be a massive and cumulative increase of nearly one-third in the long term(OECD, 2010).

The accountancy firm KPMG estimated the cost to the UK of the lowest 6% in terms of lost direct and indirect taxes, unemployment benefits, justice costs, and additional educational costs, was £2.4 *billion* per year (Gross et al., 2009). However,

> On the basis of a 79% success rate and a unit cost of £2,600 per person, we estimate that annual savings of £1.6 billion would be made as a result of providing effective numeracy intervention at the age of seven to all of the 35,843 pupils who currently leave primary school each year with very low numeracy skills.

KPMG reckons that every pound spent on intervention for the lowest 6% would generate a return of £12–19! Impressive argument.

Now many of the lowest 6%, perhaps most of them, will be dyscalculic. We know this from the best prevalence estimate – 3.4% (Reigosa-Crespo et al., 2012). So why does the UK government neglect dyscalculia? I don't know, but one some possible reason is that there are no parent-initiated organizations (comparable with the British Dyslexia Association or the National Autistic Society) to lobby government. It is not recognised by the NHS (National Health Service) while ADHD, for example, is.

This raises the question of why there is no parent-initiated organisation to lobby government for help with the offspring. Again, there doesn't appear to be research on this, but here are possible reasons:

- Lack of recognition by teachers who are not taught about dyscalculia.
- Lack of recognition by psychology professionals who are not taught about dyscalculia and the appropriate assessments and specialized interventions.
- No media campaign fronted by celebrities to make the case.
- Lack of recognition by parents and carers who have not heard about dyscalculia and so will have problems requesting assessments or specialized interventions.
- It is considered OK to be "crap at maths" in a way it isn't to be crap at reading and writing, because maths is meant to be hard and reading is not.
- Maths is a proxy for intelligence, so people who are really bad at it, must be stupid. Incidentally, the DSM IV criterion for its version of dyscalculia is a significant difference between a maths score and an IQ score: that is, low IQ is a sufficient cause of low maths (see Chapter 1).
- The problem of "labelling". Many teachers, and others, think it is bad to label children, because labels stick and children change.
- The problem of testing. Pauline Clayton, the principal tutor in maths at the Dyslexia Institute, asserts that "Good teachers get a gut feeling about their children, they know those who are underachieving," she said. "Greater awareness of dyscalculia is needed but I don't think we should go down the route of testing" (www.telegraph.co.uk/news/science/science-news/3293562/Schools-will-test-for-genetic-number-blindness.html). How reliable and valid is the teacher's gut.
- There is no agreed set of criteria for identifying dyscalculics, and no evaluated interventions, so there's no point in recognising it.
- No evidence of dyscalculia having an impact on classroom behaviour. Also, unlike dyslexia there is less evidence of dyscalculia preventing access to other curriculum areas.

In Chapters 1 and 9, I outlined various official and professional criteria currently deployed for identifying children and adults with specific learning disabilities in mathematics (the word 'dyscalculia' is rarely mentioned). In some, like DSM IV, low IQ is a disqualification for this disability. The others rely on qualitative criteria such as persistent failure to respond to intervention, or the

DfES criterion above. The US Department of Education mentions but does not define dyscalculia.

It would clearly help if there were agreed criteria for identifying dyscalculia, and it would be even more helpful if identification could lead to effective intervention. That is, science has to come up with the answers.

Science

This is where people like me come in. What science should provide is a *reliable* test of individual differences that distinguishes dyscalculia from other causes of poor or very poor numerical abilities. What do I mean by "reliable"? The most obvious and most fundamental way in which a test is reliable is that the same person will score the same each time he or she is tested. This is called "test-retest reliability". It should also be a *stable* marker of individual differences. That is, it should pick out the same group of individuals as dyscalculic if the same test is applied at different ages. Since children, even dyscalculic children improve with age, their scores on a test will also improve, so a dyscalculic child at ten may look like a typical child at five as indeed is the case in some tests(Piazza et al., 2010). Piazza et al used a "cross-sectional" study in which individuals of different ages were tested. A longitudinal study, by contrast, tests the same children at different ages. Since the child improves from year to year, the question becomes is the child still worse (or better) than his or her peers. In our study over five years, the child in lowest performing group in kindergarten was very likely to be in the lowest performing group at ten years (Reeve et al., 2012). That means our test – timed dot enumeration - was reliable and was a stable measure of individual difference even though performance on the test improves.

Tests should also be *valid*. What do I mean by "valid"? Dyscalculia is a scientist's "construct": you cannot observe it directly, only its effects. So, it is not enough for test to be a reliable and stable measure: it should reflect the underlying theory. If the theory states that poor performance on the test is sufficient for difficulty in learning arithmetic (though not necessary for this difficulty), is this in fact the case? Will it predict children who will have difficulty learning arithmetic? Of course, there will be other learners who have trouble learning arithmetic, not all of course, since there are other reasons for a poor start in learning arithmetic such as lack numerical activities in the home (see Chapter 8).

Consider the analogy with dyslexia. There are many reasons for being a poor reader, of course, including inadequate teaching, no books at home, etc, but the core deficit for most dyslexics is linguistic, particularly being aware of the sound structure of words. This is easy to test by asking them whether two words rhyme, or whether they start with the same sound (Snowling, 2000). These tests also indicate the kind of intervention that should help these children: training with rhymes and word onsets (Bradley & Bryant, 1978).

Similarly, a theory of dyscalculia should predict what kinds of *intervention* will be most effective. If the core deficit is with sets and their numerosities, training with sets should help (see Chapter 10).

Validity can also be evaluated in reference to quite different types of evidence. For example, does the test predict brain structure and function in the appropriate ways, such as in the intraparietal sulcus and in the connections from the parietal lobes to the frontal lobes? Is test performance heritable? That is, will a twin study show greater concordance between monozygotic co-twins than between dizygotic? Does it run in families as it does in dyslexia?

Heterogeneity

One practical problem with this account is that each dyscalculic is different, with a different mix of strengths and weaknesses. This will be due to differences in domain-general cognitive factors, such as working memory and spatial abilities (Rubinsten & Henik, 2009), as well as differences in family environment. This will be more pronounced when the criterion is performance on a standardized test of arithmetic rather than a test of core capacity because more cognitive and environmental factors come into play in arithmetic.

Continuum

One question that often arises is whether dyscalculia is all or none, or a continuum. That is, can one be more or less dyscalculic? I don't know the answer to this. My experience is that the severity of the arithmetical disability depends on the type of help received, on determination to improve and perhaps on the strength of domain-general cognitive capacities.

The take-home message is that wider recognition among parents and teachers requires a reliable and valid test, preferably a simple and comprehensible one, that identifies dyscalculic learners so that an appropriate individual education plan can be provided.

Now the tests I advocate in Chapter 9 may not be the most reliable and the most valid, though I believe they are the best available at the moment. It is always possible to improve them.

What can be done?

Science

To improve the science takes time and funding. There are still many important questions to answer. Here are some of the cognitive and behavioural issues that merit further research:

- For example, we need to evaluate different methods of measuring individual differences in core capacity, and the long-term stability of these measures. That is, if you are of type A when you're five years old, are you still type A at 11, at 16 at 25? This is a long-term and expensive project.

■ Are the proposed measures equally reliable and valid for different economic, social, linguistic and ethnic groups? Do they work as well in the USA as in Mexico, or China?

■ We need to look at false positive and false negative rates of different tests. A false positive diagnosis (looks dyscalculic but isn't) incurs an unnecessary cost; but a false negative diagnosis means that the learner will not get the help needed and may be handicapped for life.

■ How do differences in core capacities interact with other cognitive capacities? For example, does a small working memory capacity hinder a dyscalculic more than a typical developer?

■ What are the most effective ways of helping dyscalculics? Do these follow from the theory? And, what role can digital technologies play in this.

We still have broad-brush accounts of the relationship between dyscalculia and the brain in terms of both structure and functioning. We know a little about grey matter differences in the parietal lobes, and something about the role of the frontal lobes in typical developers, but very little about the relationship of the parietal lobes and the frontal lobes in dyscalculics. There is also very little research on the effects of different types of intervention on the brain.

■ How does learning affect the brain of dyscalculics, and is this different from the way learning affects typical developers?

■ How do different teaching methods – for example, rote learning vs conceptual learning - affect the brain?

A better understanding of the brain may also help to identify abnormalities in the very young long before they go to school. We know infants even in the first few months of life are responsive to numerosities in their environment, and these have distinctive neural signals (e.g. Izard et al., 2008). So, it may in time be possible to identify infants with different signals, which could be linked to dyscalculia. This would mean that the child starting school or in the early years would not have to suffer in classes where he or she was the only one who could not understand what the teacher was saying about numbers. It has been shown that it is possible in dyslexia to make early risk assessments using neural signals (Leppänen et al., 2002), so it should also be possible for dyscalculia.

■ Can risk of dyscalculia be identified in the infant brain?

Although we know that dyscalculia is in many cases inherited, we do not know which genes are involved. Variants of several candidate genes have been proposed but without reliable replication. Again, if we could identify these variants we might be able to spot children at risk of trouble later on and save them unnecessary suffering.

- Is it possible to identify the gene or genes responsible for dyscalculia?
- Can animal models help to find or test candidate genes?

Recognition

We have a good way of testing for the core deficit in dyscalculia, even though, as I suggested above, this can be improved. Having good ways of assessing dyscalculia is necessary, but it is not sufficient. People have to know about it. We can't rely on politicians to search out the evidence and argue for policy on its basis. They have to cajoled, threatened or encouraged.

If teachers and other professionals are not taught about dyscalculia, it is really a matter of luck whether they know about it or not. This is even more true of parents. A big media campaign that involves celebrities would help raise its profile, as has done for other neurodevelopmental disorders such as autism and dyslexia.

Even if people have heard of dyscalculia, how do they persuade governments and educational authorities to take it seriously?

- Make reference to practices or laws in other countries, such as IDEA in the US, or the Department of Education and Skills in Ireland.

It is unclear how practical this strategy is, since knowledge of these other systems is key, and this means media presence and campaigning. Social media deals with it, and there are now many websites that can be accessed with a simple search.

We need a media campaign led by worried or even angry parents demanding that something be done. Start a British Dyscalculia Association to do this.

Training professionals

This is a key issue. Dyscalculia, as I mentioned, is not widely taught to relevant professionals, though there are post-graduate courses at Bath Spa and Edge Hill Universities. The British Dyslexia Association validates courses that qualify participants to assess and support dyscalculics.

- Dyscalculia to be included in initial training for teachers, so teachers are as aware of the condition as they are of dyslexia or autism.
- Dyscalculia to be included on courses for educational, clinical, and occupational psychologists and neuropsychologists. These are often the professionals carrying out the assessment that leads to provision of additional resources and accommodations.
- Dyscalculia to be included in courses for speech and language therapists. These will often be the professionals of first recourse if the child has dyslexia or a language difficulty, which often co-occur with numeracy problems (see

Chapter 9). Some of the very best and most influential special needs teachers for dyscalculia, such as Jane Emerson, started as speech therapists.

- Dyscalculia to be included in training for special needs teachers.
- More continuing professional development courses on dyscalculia would be helpful.
- Online courses or MOOCs (Massive Open Online Courses) could be an important resource not restricted by place that could supplement the courses mentioned above.

Government policy

Governments can take the lead in recognizing dyscalculia, and making policies to identify and help dyscalculics. Though it seems rare for them to do so. In the UK, policy change will be needed.

It is not clear where ministers get their ideas for educational change. For example, the schools minister, Nick Gibb, in the current UK introduced a new test in February 2018. I quote here from the ministry's website:

> From June 2020, all pupils at the end of year 4 [8 to 9 year olds] in England will take an online multiplication tables check (MTC).
>
> The national curriculum specifies that pupils at this stage should be able to recall the multiplication tables up to and including 12x12.
>
> The check aims to support pupils to master multiplication skills, which are essential for future success in mathematics. It will help to identify pupils who have not yet mastered this mathematical concept, so additional support can be provided.
>
> (www.gov.uk/guidance/multiplication-tables-check-development-process)

I assume that Gibb was encouraged by someone that being able to recite tables was important for mathematical development. His analogy was with teaching phonics in school as a basis for skilled reading. However, with phonics there was 30 years of serious research on which to base the policy. There is no evidence that mastering the tables improves arithmetical competence, or that it is essential for future success in mathematics. (I have met distinguished mathematicians who seemed not to know their tables.) In fact, there is persuasive evidence from neurological patients that knowledge of the tables and understanding basic arithmetic are dissociable. Thus, one patient, JG (see Chapter 7), was able to recite her tables but had very poor understanding of the principles of addition and subtraction, and two patients reported by French scientists Stanislas Dehaene and Laurent Cohen also showed comparable dissociations between rote knowledge and understanding. They conclude that one neural network "contributes to the storage and retrieval of rote verbal arithmetic facts" and another to arithmetical understanding (Dehaene & Cohen, 1997).

Those failing to "master" the tables will be provided with "additional support". Nothing is said about what this support will be. Presumably, more tables training. No information is provided.

Is failing to master your tables a handicap? It seems to be no bar to becoming a minister in the Department for Education. When he announced this policy on TV, interviewers asked Gibb to do the kind of thing he is requiring of eight-year-olds. He refused to answer one interviewer's question "What's eight times nine?", and refused another interviewer's request to recite his tables (www.standard. co.uk/news/education/minister-nick-gibb-refuses-to-answer-times-tables-questions-as-he-launches-news-times-tables-policy-a3766061.html).

A previous UK Labour government produced many guidance documents about dyscalculia. These can no longer be accessed. However, the relevant material hasn't entirely disappeared. I found one on the National Centre for Excellence in the Teaching of Mathematics website.

The NCETM doesn't have anything of its own about dyscalculia, but it does or did provide a forum for anxious teachers to discuss problems with their dyscalculic pupils. However, there was an excellent document produced by the North Somerset Council about assessment and intervention. It says,

> North Somerset is committed to supporting pupils with SpLD (dyscalculia) by promoting the model "the circles of inclusion" (reproduced on P5) used in the Primary National Strategy "Learning and teaching for dyslexic children" DfES (1184–2005 CDI).

Needless to say, this document is longer available on the North Somerset website, and the relevant documents from the previous government are not even available as archived material (www.ncetm.org.uk/public/files/20535945/guidance_dyscalculia.pdf).

A previous Labour government also commissioned a report from the distinguished Oxford academic, Ann Dowker. It is entitled *What Works for Children with Mathematical Difficulties?* You may still be able to access this on The National Archives at http://webarchive.nationalarchives.gov.uk/20110202102730 or http://nationalstrategies.standards.dcsf.gov.uk/node/174504

This is a systematic and sophisticated review of arithmetic and its difficulties more broadly, but with specific comments on dyscalculia. Dr Dowker notes, quite correctly, that dyscalculics "be identified as having difficulties early on, so as to reduce the risks of intellectual confusion and emotional frustration and possibly humiliation if they are expected to cope with the typical school arithmetic curriculum without special help" (Dowker, 2009, p. 14).

To get change at the level of government policy will clearly be difficult. However, it is easy to see what is required:

- Official recognition of dyscalculia by the relevant government department (in the UK, the Department for Education) that dyscalculia (preferably by name) qualifies as a special educational need.

■ Government provides resources to schools or local education authorities for assessment and intervention. KPMG reckoned that this would cost about £2,600 per child which should be provided by government. In other countries, the cost would be different.

Summary

■ Dyscalculia is not always widely recognized by professionals, parents and governments

■ Where it is not recognized, governments do not provide the resources necessary for assessments and interventions

■ Science can provide better tools for assessment and intervention, but this requires funding and commitment

■ Better tools can help make dyscalculia more widely recognized, especially by parent organizations

■ Wider recognition can encourage government policy to change

References

Beddington, J., Cooper, C., Field, J., Goswami, U. P., Jenkins, R., & Sahakian, B. (Eds). (2008). *Foresight Mental Capital and Wellbeing Project: Final Project Report*. London: Government Office for Science.

Bradley, L., & Bryant, P. E. (1978). Difficulties in auditory organisation as a possible cause of reading backwardness. *Nature*, 271, 746–747.

Bynner, J., & Parsons, S. (1997). *Does Numeracy Matter?* London: The Basic Skills Agency.

Bynner, J., & Parsons, S. (2006). New Light on Literacy and Numeracy. Retrieved from: www.nrdc.org.uk/?p=317

Cockcroft, W. H. (1982). *Mathematics Counts: Report of the Committee of Inquiry into the Teaching of Mathematics in Schools under the Chairmanship of Dr W H Cockcroft*. London: HMSO.

Cross, C. T., Woods, T. A., & Schweingruber, H. (Eds). (2009). *Mathematics Learning in Early Childhood: Paths Toward Excellence and Equity*. Washington, DC: The National Academies Press.

Dehaene, S., & Cohen, L. (1997). Cerebral pathways for calculation: Double dissociation between rote verbal and quantitative knowledge of arithmetic. *Cortex*, 33(2), 219–250.

DfES. (2001). *Guidance to support pupils with dyslexia and dyscalculia* (DfES 0512/2001). Retrieved from: http://webarchive.nationalarchives.gov.uk/20060717053557 or www.dfes.gov.uk/schoolageparents/

Dowker, A. (2009). What works for children with mathematical difficulties? The effectiveness of intervention schemes. Retrieved from: http://webarchive.nationalarchives. gov.uk/20130323065803 or www.education.gov.uk/publications/eOrderingDownload/ 00086-2009-maths_difficulties.pdf

Gross, J., Hudson, C., & Price, D. (2009). The long term costs of numeracy difficulties. Retrieved from: www.everychildachancetrust.org

Izard, V., Dehaene-Lambertz, G., & Dehaene, S. (2008). Distinct cerebral pathways for object identity and number in human infants. *PLoS Biology*, 6, e11. doi: 10.1371/journal. pbio.0060011

Leppänen, P. H. T., Richardson, U., Pihko, E., Eklund, K. M., Guttorm, T. K., Aro, M., & Lyytinen, H. (2002). Brain Responses to Changes in Speech Sound Durations Differ Between Infants With and Without Familial Risk for Dyslexia. *Developmental Neuropsychology*, 22(1), 407–422. doi: 10.1207/S15326942dn2201_4

OECD. (2010). The High Cost of Low Educational Performance. The Long-run economic impact of improving educational outcomes. Retrieved from

Parsons, S., & Bynner, J. (2005). *Does Numeracy Matter More?* London: National Research and Development Centre for Adult Literacy and Numeracy, Institute of Education.

Piazza, M., Facoetti, A., Trussardi, A. N., Berteletti, I., Conte, S., Lucangeli, D., Dehaene, S., & Zorzi, M. (2010). Developmental trajectory of number acuity reveals a severe impairment in developmental dyscalculia. *Cognition*, 116(1), 33–41.

Reeve, R., Reynolds, F., Humberstone, J., & Butterworth, B. (2012). Stability and Change in Markers of Core Numerical Competencies. *Journal of Experimental Psychology: General*, 141(4), 649–666. doi: 10.1037/a0027520

Reigosa-Crespo, V., Valdes-Sosa, M., Butterworth, B., Estevez, N., Rodriguez, M., Santos, E., Torres, P., Suarez, R., & Lage, A. (2012). Basic Numerical Capacities and Prevalence of Developmental Dyscalculia: The Havana Survey. *Developmental Psychology*, 48(1), 123–135. doi: 10.1037/a0025356

Rubinsten, O., & Henik, A. (2009). Developmental dyscalculia: Heterogeneity might not mean different mechanisms. *Trends in Cognitive Sciences*, 13, 92–99. doi: 10.1016/j.tics.2008.11.002

Smith, A. (2004). *Making Mathematics Count: The Report of Professor Adrian Smith's Inquiry into Post-14 Mathematics Education* (Vol. 937764). London: The Stationery Office Limited.

Snowling, M. J. (2000). *Dyslexia*. Oxford: Blackwell.

Williams, P. (2008). *Independent review of mathematics teaching in early years settings and primary schools: Final report*. (DCSF-00433–2008). Retrieved from: http://dera.ioe.ac.uk/8365/7/Williams%20Mathematics_Redacted.pdf

Index

Page references in bold refer to tables. Page references in italics refer to figures.

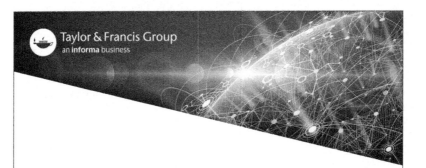

Made in the USA
Coppell, TX
29 October 2022

85412485R00111